Nutrition and Mental Health:
a handbook

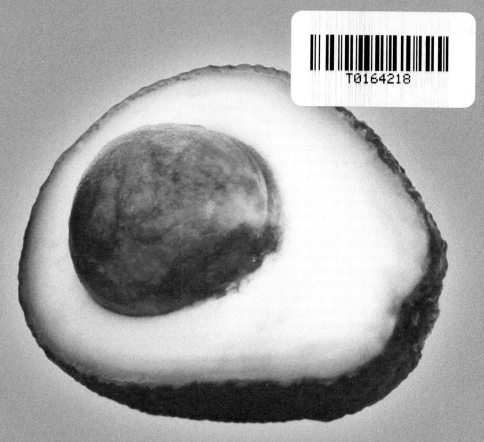

AN ESSENTIAL GUIDE TO THE RELATIONSHIP
BETWEEN DIET AND MENTAL HEALTH

Edited by Martina Watts

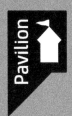

Nutrition and Mental Health: a handbook

An essential guide to the relationship between diet and mental health

Edited by Martina Watts

© Pavilion Publishing and Media Ltd, 2008, reprinted 2009; 2014.

Published by:
Pavilion Publishing and Media Ltd
Rayford House
School Road
Hove BN3 5HX
UK

Tel: +44 (0)1273 434943
Fax: +44 (0)1273 227308
Email: info@pavpub.com
Web: www.pavpub.com

The authors have asserted their rights in accordance with the *Copyright, Designs and Patents Act 1988*, to be identified as the authors of this work.

A catalogue record for this book is available from the British Library.

ISBN: 978 1 84196 245 0

Pavilion is the leading training and development provider and publisher in the health, social care and allied fields, providing a range of innovative training solutions underpinned by sound research and professional values. We aim to put our customers first, through excellent customer service and good value.

Pavilion editor: Bonnie Craig, Pavilion
Cover and page design: Faye Thompson, Pavilion
Cover photograph: Robert Owen-Wahl
Printed on paper from a sustainable resource by PrintonDemand Worldwide

Nutrition and Mental Health:

a handbook

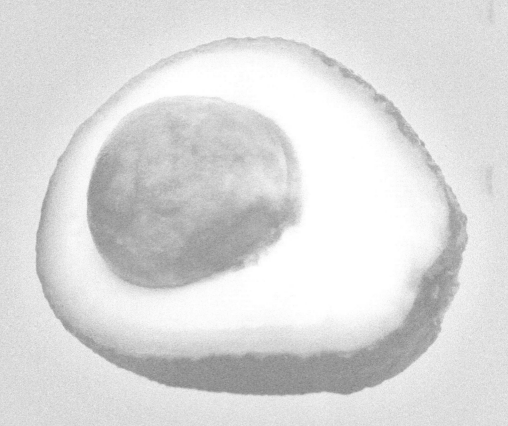

AN ESSENTIAL GUIDE TO THE RELATIONSHIP
BETWEEN DIET AND MENTAL HEALTH

Edited by Martina Watts

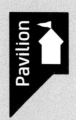

Contents

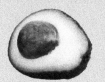

Disclaimer
This handbook aims to provide general nutritional advice but is not intended to be a substitute for professional health advice. Always consult an appropriate health professional about any specific medical problems and keep them informed of any changes.

Foreword

PROFESSOR MICHAEL A CRAWFORD

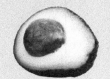

This book is about depression. Generally, we do not seem to understand the meaning of depression, unless we have suffered from it.

In 1968, when on holiday with my family, I suddenly became acutely ill with a blinding headache and temperature. '*Influenza*' said the local doctor. Quite excusable, but it became so severe, despite usual treatment for colds, that we had to abandon the holiday and my wife drove us home.

On returning home, I was severely jaundiced and running a high temperature. The diagnosis was glandular fever. The following three weeks, I suffered from deep depression the like of which is almost impossible to describe. I did not want to listen to the radio, watch television or read. All I wanted was the curtains drawn and darkness.

Recovery was slow and the treatment consisted of marmite on toast plus anti-inflammatory drugs. At least my doctor even then recognised the importance of keeping up my micronutrient status to save my brain, faced with the fact that there was little that could be done about a viral infection and that I did not want to eat. So I was fortunate to have a wise man in charge of my sickness.

What this experience made me realise was just how very serious depression is. It also made me realise that it was chemically induced by the disorder in my liver. That proved to me just how important it is to maintain a good state of nutritional chemistry for proper brain function; moreover, just how disordered blood chemistry can adversely affect the brain. This fact is so little granted, although we are currently experiencing nutritional conditions that precipitated vascular disease last century. The brain depends on good blood vessels and this is particularly important during foetal development. The placenta, which feeds the foetus, is a rapidly developing vascular system and develops before the foetal brain growth thrust in the last trimester of pregnancy.

Nutritional disorders can, of course, be induced by bad diets and in the last century we saw heart disease rise from a rarity to the number one killer. What is now happening is that brain disorders have taken over. They are now the number one burden of ill health in Europe (Andlin-Sobocki *et al*, 2005) The cost for the 25 member states at 2004 prices was 386 billion euros. Mental ill health is now spreading world wide (Global Forum for Health Research, online) and it is likely that the globalisation of Western food systems is one of the major factors in this spread.

This book brings together several authors to understand better the causes and ways of dealing with depression. With so little attention paid to nutrition and the brain, this book is timely and will make a significant contribution to the dissemination of knowledge on this misunderstood topic of depression and allied disorders of brain function.

References

Andlin-Sobocki P, Jönsson B, Wittchen H and Olesen J (2005) Cost of disorders of the brain in Europe. *European Journal of Neurology* **12** (S1) 1–27.

Global Forum for Health Research [online] available at: www.globalforumhealth.org [accessed: 30/05/08].

Editor's foreword

MARTINA WATTS

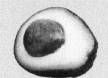

The handbook for every car manufactured will specify, quite precisely, the grade and type of engine oil that should be used in its engine. Dire warnings are presented as to the inevitable consequences if this advice is ignored, such as loss of power, excessive internal wear and tear, and risk of breakdown. The manufacturer's guarantee may be invalidated if the buyer exhibits such a degree of carelessness with their purchase. We generally accept these conditions as entirely reasonable. After all, the car was designed specifically to use particular fuels and lubricants, and surely only a fool would risk such a sizeable investment through meanness or laziness. When it comes to our own human bodies, such rationality is abandoned. We have thrown away the handbook, or simply forgotten there ever was one.

We believe that we can fuel a body and lubricate it with whatever we want, without regard to any inherent 'design constraints'. Further, we believe that there can be no adverse consequence to this behaviour, whether physical or mental. More spectacularly, we believe that as and when our bodies do break down, there cannot possibly be any link to our own consumptive habits. The very notion appears ridiculous, so instead we seek out magic bullets in the form of instant chemical remedies. Although such chemicals may be useful and necessary in some cases, antidepressants, mood stabilisers and antipsychotics also have side effects (Caplan, 2008; Rethink, 2006; Tschoner *et al*, 2007). A nutritional approach should therefore be considered at the outset.

Many health professionals are currently working to improve diet and nutrition for people with mental health problems. The themes in this book have been discussed at a series of recent Pavilion conferences that examined the link between diet, nutrition and mental health, underpinned by the latest research. Several leading health practitioners reveal their insights, clinical experiences and most successful nutritional strategies, and how to put these into practice, including Dr Abram Hoffer, a Psychiatrist who pioneered the orthomolecular treatment of schizophrenic patients as long as 50 years ago. He is still waiting to see medicine return to nutrition and nutrients. The general consensus among all co-authors is that we honour our genetic blueprint (our manufacturer's handbook) and adapt it to the climate we live in. If our dietary intake or digestion is inadequate, the broad consequences are entirely predictable.

The most effective treatment is to *combine a variety of dietary and lifestyle strategies* as described in the cases overleaf, and more independent research is required to confirm what works best for whom and when. There must now be wider recognition of the fact that people have individual nutritional and biochemical requirements and that 'one size' definitely does not 'fit all'.

> Sarah-Jane[*] (39 years old) came to see me with a diagnosis of bi-polar disorder along with depression, exhaustion and constipation. She also suffered from frequent infections, hives, hay fever, weight gain, excessive thirst and thrush. She was taking various antipsychotic medications, mood stabilisers and antidepressants and had a contraceptive implant. In all, she was taking 13 different types of drugs every day. Sarah-Jane started 'cleaning up' her diet and, with her doctor's approval, slowly reducing her drug regime. I designed a nutritional programme, which included stomach acid support, probiotics, an effective multivitamin/ mineral and high-quality essential fatty acids. In addition, we discussed ways of stabilising her blood sugar and alternatives to gluten- and casein-containing foods. We also tackled an underlying yeast infestation. Sarah-Jane was a model client with a very supportive partner, yet we had many ups and downs. At present she is off all drugs except the antidepressant and no longer requires a community psychiatric nurse. She feels healthy and is actively involved in helping her husband's business.

> Ollie[*] (23 years old) came to see me with a diagnosis of schizophrenia. He wasn't hearing voices in his head, but ethereal music. He regularly consumed alcohol, smoked cigarettes and used recreational drugs. Within six months he had weaned himself off stimulants, started eating a nutritious diet and taking a few supplements. He told me that he had improved to such an extent that he no longer heard strange music or required medication. I lost contact with Ollie, but encountered him by chance a few years later. He had not been able to stick to his healthy lifestyle, had relapsed and was back on medication.

* Names have been changed.

People with more severe mental health problems require ongoing practical and financial support to maintain an improved diet and lifestyle. Complex interactions between genes, lifestyle, diet and environment are increasingly demanding that nutrition health professionals[1] become members of the multidisciplinary team assessing patients with mental health problems.

Nutritional progress in institutions can be even more difficult to achieve, and requires committed, informed individuals willing to consistently drive through the required dietary improvements within organisations that can seem almost designed to resist change. A recurring problem is the management of conflict between 'prescribed nutrition' and 'patient choice' when such choice is based on flawed information (eg. wanting to eat cake all day). It is possible, with sound nutritional education and involvement of all parties, to challenge and ultimately change both established practices within organisations and compelling individual habits, as demonstrated in the following project.

In 2004, the Support Services Manager at a secure unit for young offenders contacted me requesting suggestions for healthier eating practices. She was aware that convenience food has adverse effects on the mood, learning and behaviour of young people, but faced considerable opposition in reducing sugar, salt, additives, refined carbohydrates and hydrogenated fats in the food at the unit.

'Unhealthy' meal choices were gradually phased out with simple, natural home-cooked meals and 'treats' were replaced with healthier alternatives within budget. Tastier main meals meant that the young people ate less sandwiches and baked goods. Cakes, biscuits and crisps were removed at break times and replaced with a variety of fresh fruit, purchased from the local market, guaranteeing fresh, seasonal and nutritious produce. Higher quality oils were used and frying restricted to chips only. Quality meat was bought from a new local meat supplier at a discount. Instead of supplying sugar bowls and salt cellars at each table, a limited amount of sugar and salt sachets were provided and controlled by staff. A healthy tuck shop offered low-fat crisps, dried fruit and selected fruit juices and confectionery without additives or artificial sweeteners.

The healthy eating project has been surprisingly cost effective. Due to less wastage, savings have been made. It takes newcomers a month to adapt and a visible change in physical appearance with less weight gain is noted. Staff confirm that bedtimes and weekends are much calmer with less aggravated behaviour. A monitoring report by the General Manager stated that 'the use of physical restraints is down by 60% from 2005/06 to 2006/07' (Watts, 2007).

Clearly, not all people with mental health or learning and behavioural problems eat junk food, have unhealthy habits or suffer from poor gut health. The complex case history of Duncan (**Chapter 8**) reveals that a virus is likely to have been an underlying factor in the development of his illness. However, nutritional therapy contributed to his recovery and alleviated many of his symptoms.

Duncan's harrowing story is of particular relevance because it exposes the struggle with entrenched institutional procedures and the discriminatory processes evident in our healthcare system. His mother demonstrated what can be achieved through tenacity and scientific curiosity by assembling a team of health professionals from a variety of disciplines and countries, working together to help her son recover. This positive spirit of scientific enquiry, which often challenges the institutional or bureaucratic status-quo, has almost been lost, but needs to be rediscovered to see us through the current crisis in mental health. It is this spirit of enterprise, combined with an abiding respect for the nutritional requirements of the human brain, which this handbook seeks to inspire in the current generation, and pass on to the next.

Endnote

[1] To distinguish between dieticians, nutritional therapists and public health nutritionists please see *Briefing Note. Understanding the differences between nutrition health professionals* at www.bant.org.uk [accessed: 30/05/08].

References

Caplan P (2008) The pills that make us fat. Psychiatric drugs are adding to the obesity epidemic. *New Scientist* **2646**.

Rethink (2006) *Side Effects of Mood Stabilisers* [online] available at: www.rethink.org/living_with_mental_illness/treatment_and_therapy/medication/ mood_stabilisers/side_effects_of.html [accessed: 30/05/08].

Tschoner A, Engl J, Laimer M, Kaser S, Rettenbacher M, Fleischhacker WW, Patsch JR and Ebenbichler CF (2007) Metabolic side effects of antipsychotic medication. *International Journal of Clinical Practice* **61** (8) 1356–1370.

Watts M (2007) Healthy eating project at Redbank Community Home. *The Nutrition Practitioner* **8** (3).

Contributors

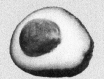

Michael Ash BSc (Hons), DO, ND, Dip ION, MIoD has been in clinical practice since 1982 as an Osteopath, Naturopath and Nutritional Therapist, and is a pioneer of functional medicine in the UK. He has developed health- and function-improving strategies for elite athletes, patients with metabolic, immune and gastrointestinal disturbances, neurodevelopmental and mental health problems, as well as other diverse conditions. Since 1999 he has researched, lectured and published on the mucosal immune system within the gastro-intestinal tract and its effect on the health of the body. During this time he has established nutrition-based immunotherapeutics and developed a special interest in patients with autism, neurodevelopmental problems, functional bowel problems and recurrent pregnancy loss associated with immune disruption. He is a Fellow of the Royal Society of Medicine and a member of the Psychoneuroimmunology Research Society, New York Academy of Sciences, and the Society of Mucosal Immunology. He is also Managing Director of Nutri-Link Ltd.

Oscar Umahro Cadogan is a recognised authority on dietary and nutritional interventions for treating disease, natural sports nutrition, product quality and functional medicine laboratory testing in Denmark. He lectures extensively to practitioners and educational institutions and is Co-editor of *The International Textbook of Functional Medicine*, a comprehensive updated textbook on functional medicine. He works as a Consultant in the health sector on research, legislation and the formulation of products and natural functional foods for the European and North American markets. He has published a range of healthy cookbooks, a book about natural treatments for serious gastrointestinal disease and is a regular contributor to both general media and professional publications in Scandinavia.

Dr Natasha Campbell-McBride MD, MMedSci, MMedSci graduated as a Medical Doctor in 1984 from Bashkir Medical University in Russia. She gained a postgraduate degree in Neurology at Moscow Medical University. After practising for five years as a Neurologist and three years as a Neurosurgeon she moved to the UK, completing a second postgraduate degree in Human Nutrition at Sheffield University. Natasha returned to practice in 2000 at the Cambridge Nutrition Clinic. She is recognised as one of the leading experts on the treatment of children and adults with learning disabilities and other mental disorders, as well as children and adults with digestive and immune disorders. Her book *Gut and Psychology Syndrome. Natural treatment of autism, ADHD, dyslexia, dyspraxia, depression and schizophrenia* explains the connection between the patient's physical state and brain function. Her new book *Put Your Heart in Your Mouth* explores the confusion surrounding nutrition and cardiovascular disease. Natasha is a keynote speaker at professional conferences around the world.

Professor Michael A Crawford PhD, CBiol, FIBiol, FRCPath is a leading expert in brain chemistry and human nutrition, specialising in dietary fats and the health benefits of essential fatty acids, in particular the physics of DHA in cell signalling. Other special themes of interest are nutrition in developing countries and applications to food and agriculture. He was Head of Department of Biochemistry and Nutrition at the Nuffield Institute of Comparative Medicine in London for 25 years and was Special Professor at the Department of Applied Biochemistry and Nutrition, University of Nottingham for 16 years. Michael is founder and Director of London's Institute of Brain Chemistry and Human Nutrition at the new London Metropolitan University. Since 1960, Michael has published three books, including *The Driving Force: Food, evolution and the future* (1989), and over 280 scientific communications. His work has also extended to the development of a new understanding of the role of nutrition in human evolution with its relevance to contemporary nutrition-related disease. He is a Consultant for WHO, FAO, Millenium Danone Chair at University of Gent; Chair at the Albert Schweitzer International University in Geneva and a member of the Department of Health Committee on Borderline Substances.

Antony J Haynes BA (Hons) Dip ION has spent 25 years researching nutrition and its impact on health. He has a Sports Science degree and a Diploma from The Institute for Optimum Nutrition (1992), and has been practising as a Nutritional Therapist since 1993. Antony has met over 10,000 patients with a wide range of health concerns. Antony has taught nutrition at the leading colleges for nutritional therapy education for 15 years. He has also taught postgraduate courses and has made over 300 presentations to interested groups. Annual trips to the US for his own continuing education have helped him to keep up to date with the fast-moving science of nutrition. Antony has written two books: *The Insulin Factor* (2004) and *The Food Intolerance Bible* (co-written, 2005). Antony is a co-founder and Technical Director of Nutri-Link Ltd.

Dr Abram Hoffer (Retired) PhD, FRCP(C), RNCP is recognised internationally for his pioneering discoveries in the field of psychiatry and medicine, teaming up with Humphrey Osmond and Linus Pauling to found orthomolecular medicine. He was born in Canada in 1917. After his early training in biochemistry and agricultural science, he specialised in psychiatry, working as Director of Psychiatric Research at the Department of Public Health, then Associate Professor (Research) Psychiatry, College of Medicine at the University of Saskatchewan. Abram and Humphrey developed the first biochemical theory of schizophrenia and co-developed the Hoffer-Osmond Diagnostic Test for schizophrenia, uncovering the connection between deficiencies in specific nutrients and mental illness. Abram, with R Altshul and J Stephen, also introduced the use of niacin as a powerful agent to lower total cholesterol and elevate HDL (high-density lipoprotein) levels in the blood. He has written over 500 papers in medical journals and has written 30 books, including *Orthomolecular Medicine for Physicians*. Abram is still in private practice as a Consultant in nutrition and the proper use of vitamins and continues to edit the *Journal of Orthomolecular Medicine*.

Dr Andrew McCulloch has been Chief Executive of the Mental Health Foundation since October 2002. Prior to this, Andrew was Director of Policy at the Sainsbury Centre for Mental Health for six years. He was formerly a Senior Civil Servant in the Department of Health for 16 years and was responsible for mental health and learning disabilities policy from 1992 to 1996. He has particular interests in policy development, partnership working, models of mental health care, human resources and public mental health. He has spoken and published widely on mental health issues. Andrew's other experience has included being a school governor, the non-executive Director of an NHS Trust, and the Chair of Mental Health Media, a charity dedicated to giving people with mental health problems and learning disabilities a voice. His PhD study related to psycho-social adjustment to old age.

Dr Brian McDonogh MBChB, BMedSci, MScNutrMed is a GP specialist in nutritional medicine with more than 25 years of experience. He practises nutritional and integrated medicine in Horsham, West Sussex, combining conventional and complementary therapies. This enables him to take a holistic approach to identifying and treating the underlying causes of ill health. He believes in giving people with chronic illness sufficient time and aims to help them achieve a feeling of being more in control of their illness. This involves good history taking, physical examination, appropriate investigation and improving insight into the problems identified. Brian regularly lectures in his specialist field to university and college students, gives talks to interested self-help groups and charities and provides educational sessions for healthcare professionals.

Kate Neil MSc RN RM FRSA is Director of the Centre for Nutrition Education and Lifestyle Management (CNELM). The Centre teaches a BSc in Nutritional Therapy validated by Middlesex University and postgraduate courses accredited by Middlesex University leading to a masters degree. Kate is a Lecturer, Writer and Nutritional Therapy Practitioner. She authored *Balancing Hormones Naturally* and is founding Editor of the peer-reviewed journal *The Nutrition Practitioner*. Kate specialises in providing nutritional support for parents with children with learning and behavioural difficulties and women's health from pre-conceptual care to menopause and beyond. Kate has been committed to improving educational training standards since 1987. She directed the Institute for Optimum Nutrition for several years and was part of the team to develop and implement the first BSc Nutritional Therapy degree course at the University of Westminster. Kate is Clinical Supervisor for the team of nutritional therapists at Penny Brohn Cancer Care and is an expert adviser for several companies in the industry. Kate received the 2004 Natural Trade Show Award for Outstanding Contribution to the Nutritional Therapy Community.

Jane Nodder trained as a Nutritional Therapist at the Institute of Optimum Nutrition in Putney, following a management career in business. She has a nutrition practice in London and works as a Lecturer and Clinic Supervisor for the BSc Nutritional Therapy degree course at the University of Westminster, London. Jane is currently studying for a MSc in Nutritional Medicine at the University of Surrey, Guildford. She is a member of the British Association for Applied Nutrition and Nutritional Therapy (BANT) and sits on its ethics committee. Jane's areas of special interest include eating disorders and weight management, endocrine function and mental health. She was a member of the NICE Guideline Development Group for Eating Disorders (2002–2004) and delivers training for a range of groups to raise awareness about eating disorders. Through her company, Nutriworks Ltd, Jane runs nutrition workshops and seminars for healthcare professionals, businesses and the public both in the UK and in France.

Dr Alexandra J Richardson DPhil(Oxon), PGCE is a founding Director of the UK charity Food and Behaviour Research (www.fabresearch.org), a visiting Research Fellow at the Universities of Oxford and Bristol and a leading expert on the role of omega-3 fatty acids in behaviour, learning and mood. She carried out the first controlled treatment trials of omega-3 for behaviour and learning in relation to ADHD, dyslexia and dyspraxia, played a key role in early research into omega-3 for adult psychiatric disorders and currently has more than 80 research publications in peer-reviewed journals and academic books. Her ongoing research includes experimental studies and controlled nutritional treatment trials in both children and adults, and collaborations on two large-scale European research programmes investigating the genetics of neurodevelopmental disorders and their epidemiology. Alex is also the author of *They Are What You Feed Them* (Harper Thorson, 2006), which provides practical dietary advice and a uniquely accessible summary of the scientific evidence that nutrition affects children's mental development and performance, with all author royalties dedicated to the Food and Behaviour Research charity.

Tara St John is Policy Officer at the Mental Health Foundation. She was involved in the Mental Health Foundation's Feeding Minds campaign and has been interested in the role that diet plays in mental health and well-being since first exploring non-medical alternatives to overcome her own experience of depression.

Professor Vera Stejskal PhD is Associate Professor of Immunology, University of Stockholm, Sweden and First Medical Faculty at Charles University, Prague, Czech Republic. After the Russian invasion of Czechoslovakia in August 1968, she left the country to live in Sweden with her family. She worked at the Department of Immunology at the University of Stockholm where she became Associate Professor of Immunology in 1976. In 1978 she became the Director of the Department of Immunotoxicology at Astra Pharmaceuticals, where she developed the MELISA® test for testing of Type IV allergies. Vera has been affiliated with the Department of Clinical Chemistry, Danderyd's Hospital and the Karolinska

Institute in Stockholm, Sweden. Currently she is working part time at the Department of Immunology and Microbiology, First Medical Faculty at Charles University where she teaches and continues her research on the effect of metals and diseases. She is an adviser to the World Health Organization, a frequent lecturer at major conferences around the world, the author of more than 100 scientific publications and the owner of MELISA® patent and trademark.

Caroline Stokes MMedSci, BSc is a Nutrition Scientist with the British Nutrition Foundation (BNF) in London, where her current work focuses on the dissemination and communication of evidence-based nutrition science. She has a Masters of Medical Science degree in Human Nutrition from the University of Sheffield and a BSc degree in Psychology. Prior to working with the BNF, Caroline held research appointments with the Medical Research Council's Human Nutrition Research in Cambridge and with the Doncaster and South Humber Healthcare NHS Trust. In her research, Caroline has made significant contributions to investigating the relation of nutrition and mental health, in particular on dietary interventions for the treatment of depression and schizophrenia. She has also published and lectured extensively in many other areas of nutrition science.

Dr David Thomas DC initially graduated in Geology and later gained an MSc in Mineral Exploration from Imperial College. He worked for nine years in copper, cobalt, lead, zinc, gold and uranium exploration and mining, and during this period was elected as a Fellow of the Geological Society. David subsequently retrained in the US as a Chiropractor and established his practice in Forest Row, East Sussex in 1982. He later incorporated nutritional therapy into his practice and is a founding member of the Register of Nutritional Therapists. This background has provided him with an unusual insight to the origin, therapeutic uses and toxic potential of minerals and trace elements. In 2002, David conducted his initial research work into the historical loss of minerals and trace elements in the food available to us as a nation. This research work has recently been updated.

Laurie Trott PhD, Msc, BA (Hons) CACPD has studied for many years in the field of discrimination and culture. He is former Managing Director and Chief Consultant of Equilibra, a company specialising in identifying and tackling institutionalised discrimination. He is acknowledged as a leading authority on this subject. Over the past five years, Laurie has examined the relationship between current medical practice and other forms of (so called) alternative therapy and has formed strong conclusions about the inadequacies of the current predominant medical paradigm operating in the UK. Laurie has trained a substantial number of psychiatrists and psychiatric staff in tackling institutional discrimination in a number of health authorities across the country.

Linda Trott has been studying nutrition and complementary medicine since the birth of her first child in 1979. She is a qualified Aromatherapist, Reflexologist and Remedial Masseuse. She worked extensively with her husband, helping to run

Equilibra and assisting a number of high-profile research projects as Research Manager. Linda has recently been instrumental in bringing together therapists and experts in a variety of fields to enable them to work together to treat the individual needs of patients and find holistic solutions for them. Linda has a lifelong passion for animals and is founder and President of the Pinoso Association for the Protection of Animals in Spain.

Martina Watts BA (Hons) Dip ION is a BANT-registered Nutritional Therapist with special experience working with children and adults suffering from digestive, behavioural and immune problems. Her interest in human nutrition began after both her children were diagnosed with severe multiple allergies. Martina runs a private practice in Brighton and works as an independent Nutrition Consultant for schools, local government and Nuffield Proactive Health. Martina has convened five Pavilion conferences examining the increasing impact of our technological age on diet, the established links with physical and mental health problems, and how these trends can be reversed. She is currently on the MSc Nutritional Medicine programme at Surrey University. Martina is a member of the Guild of Health Writers and has been a regular newspaper columnist since 1999.

Introduction

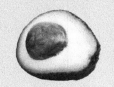

DR ANDREW MCCULLOCH
CHIEF EXECUTIVE, MENTAL HEALTH FOUNDATION

TARA ST JOHN
POLICY OFFICER, MENTAL HEALTH FOUNDATION

The profound relationship between diet and health (physical and mental) has been remarked on since ancient times. Greek and Chinese medicine, for example, both posit inter-relationships between diet and the processing of nutrients and mood, well-being, temperament and mental disorder, all mediated by biological and familial factors. In terms of the development of modern health care, diet has remained important, but we have perhaps lost the sense of the centrality of nutrition to human health and well-being. Specifically, we seem to have lost any sense that diet may be closely related to mental health (McCulloch and Ryrie, 2006; Mental Health Foundation, 2006).

Recent context

Much has been said and done in recent years in relation to the benefits of a healthy diet and good nutrition, however mental health has not been explicitly linked in to this at a national level. There is a pressing need for government to include mental health and well-being in public health messages about good nutrition, and for the health service to understand the important relationship between diet and mental health and to incorporate this into care planning and delivery. This book will help us to do this.

Over the last five to 10 years there has been a significant increase in our national focus on food – where it comes from, how it is modified, what is added to it, organic versus non-organic farming methods, and most recently an awareness of the damaging environmental effect of 'food miles'. Alongside this growing interest in production, there has been a concurrent increased focus on the role played by diet in health and disease. As a society we are becoming more aware of the detrimental effect of a poor diet on our health and of the protective role of a healthy diet.

This growing 'food consciousness' is due to a range of factors, but the growing prevalence of obesity among adults and children, and of the diseases associated with obesity, is key. In its 2004 report on obesity, The House of Commons Health Committee reviewed current policy determinants affecting the rise in obesity, and concluded that national food and health policy lacked coherence, integration and effectiveness (House of Commons Health Committee, 2004). In May 2007, The European Commission published a white paper outlining a strategy on nutrition and obesity-related issues (Commission of the European Communities, 2007).

Other factors in our growing consciousness include:

- the financial burden to the health service
- a desire to 'reconnect' with nature and for food to be as natural as possible
- the desire to remain 'biologically young' for as long as possible
- significant evidence of the central role of nutrition in foetal development and in children's physical and mental growth.

Awareness about healthy diets has been raised through television series such as Jamie Oliver's *School Dinners* and a host of other programmes. At the same time, the government has produced a number of public health initiatives such as the 'five-a-day' campaign and *Choosing Health* (Department of Health, 2004) in a tentative step towards health promotion. As a result, the food industry has had to adapt. The big supermarkets have introduced 'healthy option' ranges, organically produced and locally sourced merchandise, and labelling showing nutrient/fat content and country of origin and so on.

However, despite the growing awareness of the central importance of food to health and well-being, there has been little focus on the links between food and mental health. In *Choosing Health*, both diet and mental health are acknowledged as being central to overall well-being but the link is not made between the two. Nor is it made in the more recent nutritional action plans and guidance. This perhaps reflects the ignorance of most public health practitioners about the key importance of mental health to public health.

There has, however, been some recent interest in the link between diet and behaviour. The Associate Parliamentary Food and Health Forum have very recently published a report on the influence of nutrition on mental health (2008). The report presents a strong case for the relationship between diet and mental health and summarises key factors thought to be beneficial to mental health and behaviour based on evidence to date. It states, however, that there is a dearth of research in this area and that a great deal more investigation is needed. The report makes 19 recommendations covering areas such as:

- Department of Health messages on a healthy diet should emphasise the importance of a balanced diet for optimum mental, as well as physical, health
- government should commission research on food and mental health
- further work to clarify the role of essential fatty acids (EFAs) and oily fish
- training is required for GPs and other medical professionals
- more dieticians are required
- NHS trusts should carry out a nutritional assessment of people presenting with mental health problems such as depression or symptoms of psychosis
- nutritional trials for young offenders should be made a priority given the high risk of self-harm and suicide
- public health initiatives should encourage people to eat oily fish.

Programmes of treatment based on the association between diet and mental health are occurring sporadically within the NHS as a result of individual provider initiatives. For example, the Doncaster and South Humber Trust Food and Mood Clinic, and the Leicestershire NHS Nutrition and Dietetic Service, have strong food and public health awareness elements, as well as nutritional screening for people with mental health problems and learning disabilities. Support and training is also provided for mental health practitioners on diet and mental health and learning disabilities. However, *'nutrition is still a Cinderella subject within NHS'* (Rex, 2007).

Mental health and diet – why are they related?

While not taking a reductionist approach, it must be assumed that a healthy brain and nervous system is the platform for good mental health and that at least some of the effects of diet (good or bad) on mental health will be mediated by the effects of nutrients on the brain. However, there may also be indirect effects via social and psychological mechanisms.

Many of the impacts that diet may have on mental health, of course, mirror impacts on physical health because of the interdependence of the central nervous system (CNS), and cardiovascular, immune and endocrine systems. This interdependence presumably reflects observed correlations, for example, between cardiovascular disease, depression and type 2 diabetes. However, of the major known influences on mental health, such as activity levels and employment status, diet is one of the less well understood because of the dearth of thinking and gold standard research on this issue during the 20th century. However, this evidence base is growing as reflected in this timely book. This evidence base relates mainly to the dietary factors that might treat, prevent or cause mental illnesses, but we can also begin to make assumptions about the 'mentally healthy' diet.

The possible relationships between diet and mental health and mental illnesses

Clearly this will be complex. People do not eat in a vacuum. Diet is influenced by social, psychological and cultural issues and by the pre-existence of mental or physical disorder. Some of the possible relationships, which are not mutually exclusive, will be as follows:

- a biochemical developmental relationship in which the diet of the individual and his or her mother will affect brain development because of the impact of nutrients or their absence during crucial developmental stages. This model can equally well apply to senescence, which might not, in a strict sense, be seen as a continuation of 'development'. Some have suggested that this may be important in diseases such as schizophrenia or dementia

- recent biochemical impacts on the brain, for example, down-regulation after sugar or caffeine highs. Anecdotally, children seem to be particularly prone to these episodes and some have linked this with ADHD. Additives and pollutants may also have a role here

- poor diet could be seen as directly 'causal' in mental illness. However, poor diet will usually be a part of a complex chain or web of causation. Other common elements of this web may include income, geography, culture, upbringing, institutional history, substance misuse and physical health and activity

- poor digestive health (which itself can, of course, have biological or psychological causation or which can be related to key covariants or correlates of mental ill health) can affect whether food eaten is digested properly and whether key nutrients are absorbed

- good diet can be seen as protective of good mental health and preventative of mental illness. While, generally speaking, we could recommend a Mediterranean-style diet as protective, there will be complications. Some diets will be better than others at protecting against specific mental disorders and some individuals with, for example, metabolic disorders or learning disabilities, may require highly specific diets to help them remain mentally well

- socio-psychological aspects of our relationship with food, for example, eating in family or other groups may be more beneficial than eating alone, but this may be affected by personality and how the situation is construed by the individual or individuals involved. There is little research on this issue or other indirect relationships between diet and mental health, such as links between obesity and bullying and self-esteem, for example.

Generally speaking, these possible different relationships have not been well thought through, and most of the research so far has adopted a simplistic causal model between the absence or presence of dietary components and certain mental illnesses. However, it is important that individual contributions on this issue are understood in this wider context. It is clear that these different variables will interact dynamically over time – a simple cause and effect model is rarely very robust in mental health (Friedli, 2008).

What have we learned so far?

While much of the relationship between mental health and diet is unclear in public health terms, we already know enough to promote a Mediterranean-style diet both for mental and physical health reasons. We also have enough evidence to justify public policies that promote mentally healthy diets in children and pregnant women, as the long-term damage of unhealthy eating may impact more on the developing brain. We need to be clear that the absence of gold standard research on the links between specific mental illnesses and treatments does not mean that we do not have a sufficiently clear case for public health measures that can *at worst* do no harm or produce generalised health improvements without reducing mental illness as such.

Once we, again, recognise that diet is one of the fundamental cornerstones of good mental health, significant practice implications emerge. These include:

■ ensuring that diet is part of an overall lifestyle assessment for people with mental illness, which also includes issues such as physical activity, relationships and substance misuse

■ ensuring that primary and secondary care services can routinely provide dietary advice

■ developing more treatment and health promotion services for key groups who may benefit, such as people with depression who do not respond to antidepressants and people on atypical (newer) antipsychotics that can lead to weight gain

■ understanding that diet can underpin other approaches to treatment, especially medication and exercise.

I hope this introduction has been helpful in beginning to sketch out the complex and dynamic relationship between mental health and diet where mental health and mental illness related factors, dietary factors and other biological, psychological and social factors interact in a dynamic way over time. The co-authors of this book are hugely experienced nutrition practitioners working in direct patient care and give practical guidance on the main issues known so far in this rapidly developing field.

While the authors of this book, and indeed the Mental Health Foundation, are dedicated to getting good-quality information to the general public, this is no easy task in mental health as evidenced in the recent publicity about antidepressants. Caution is always needed in considering any changes to one's own or a loved one's medication, diet and supplements and it is imperative to discuss changes with a GP and suitably qualified health practitioners. Whatever the future holds, we are already clear that reactions to diet, supplements or medication regimes are partly individually determined.

References

Associate Parliamentary Food and Health Forum (2008) *The Links between Diet and Behaviour: The influence of nutrition on mental health.* London: Associate Parliamentary Food and Health Forum.

Commission of the European Communities (2007) *A Strategy for Europe on Nutrition, Overweight and Obesity-related Health Issues.* Brussels: European Commission.

Department of Health (2004) *Choosing Health.* London: The Stationery Office.

Friedli L (2008) *Understanding Mental Health as a Determinant of Health and Social Outcomes.* London and Copenhagen: Mental Health Foundation and The World Health Organization.

House of Commons Health Committee (2004) *Obesity.* London: The Stationery Office.

McCulloch A and Ryrie I (2006) The impact of diet on mental health. *Mental Health Review* **11** (4) 19–22.

Mental Health Foundation (2006) *Feeding Minds: The impact of food on mental health.* London: Mental Health Foundation.

Rex D (2007) NHS prescribing drugs 'when diet might help children with autism'. *Sunday Herald* 7 January (David Rex, lead child health dietician with NHS Highland quoted).

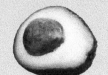

Chapter 1
Modern diets: a recipe for madness
OSCAR UMAHRO CADOGAN

What we eat was not meant for man nor beast

Mankind was 'raised' on food that differs very much from our modern diet. In a review article on nutrition and health published in *The American Journal of Clinical Nutrition* in 2005, Cordain *et al* state: '*The evolutionary collision of our ancient genome with the nutritional qualities of recently introduced foods may underlie many of the chronic diseases of Western civilization.*' In other words, modern refined foods are not 'compatible' with the human race, as they are so dissimilar to the foods and diets that we have thrived on for most of our evolutionary history. This mismatch between needs and sustenance leads to dysfunction that is expressed as diseases of civilisation, health problems in general and premature ageing. Eating modern refined foods – using the wrong kind of fuel – leads to less than optimum physical and mental functioning in the short term and sets the stage for the development of diseases of civilisation in the long term.

With the emerging acceptance that mental disorders and mental dysfunction are also to be considered among the diseases of civilisation, it should come as no surprise that modern diets are also one of the major culprits when it comes to the massive increase in the incidence of developmental, learning and behavioural disorders, as well as mental and psychiatric problems that we experience in modern societies. Autism, Asperger's syndrome, dyslexia, dyspraxia, attention deficit disorder (ADD), attention deficit hyperactivity disorder (ADHD) and similar disorders are very much about nutrition, or rather the lack of nutrition, in modern foods. These problems are not simply hardwired into our brains from birth or exclusively caused by external events, although genetic heritage and upbringing also play a role. Nor is the increased prevalence of such disorders simply due to us being better at diagnosing. Modern food really is a recipe for madness, especially for those who are genetically susceptible and those subjected to excessive stress, sadness and neglect.

Our Paleolithic heritage

There are several major differences between the foods and diets that mankind has subsisted on for most of our evolutionary history and our modern diets. A major and significant difference is the fact that mankind was reared on 'whole' and 'unrefined' foods. Our body is naturally adapted to foods and a diet with such characteristics. Irrespective of which region of the world, which environment, which time period and which population you look at, the foods eaten were 'whole' and 'unrefined' in the sense that:

- they had a high nutrient density (ie. more fibre, vitamins, minerals, antioxidants, phytochemicals, polyunsaturated fatty acids and amino acids per calorie)

- they had grown or developed in their natural environment (animals, birds and insects were outside, physically active and eating the foods that they were designed for; crops grew in soil and climates that allowed their growth without aids such as fertilisers and pesticides)

- the changes and alterations made to foods during preparation were minor compared with current practice

- the release of energy into the bloodstream following ingestion was generally much slower than the rate at which energy is released from modern foods

- food required significant physical activity, time and energy to obtain, prepare, ingest and digest compared with modern food – consider the fact that you can ingest sufficient calories for most of the day in less than 10 minutes at a fast-food restaurant without any significant effort on your part

- the amount and rate of new constituents found in foods in previous centuries was relatively low compared with the rate of introduction of new constituents in modern societies (consider the thousands of chemicals introduced into our environment and the thousands of new constituents in foods created by modern processing and additives in the last 100 years).

Modern foods are in some respects as alien to the human body as petrol is to a diesel engine; as inappropriate for sustenance as a tiger would find grass, or a horse would find meat. The reason that we, as a species, are not dying is because the human body is both resilient and flexible – it makes compromises to survive. If our diet is substandard, we specifically decrease the energy and resources allocated to 'non-essential-to-survival' issues, such as the finer aspects of brain functioning. Depression, dyslexia or hyperactivity will not kill you outright or prevent you from having children, nor will cardiovascular disease or obesity. So, despite eating a diet and living a lifestyle that is detrimental, we survive, albeit at a cost to our well-being and sanity.

Characteristics of modern foods and diets

Modern diets and the refined foods that make up the majority of what we ingest have several characteristics.

1. A high glycaemic load due to the presence of refined sugars and grain products, particularly refined grain products, and a rapid release of contained energy.

2. A high concentration of long-chain saturated fats compared with other types of fats in animal products derived from conventionally raised poultry, pigs and cattle.

3. A relatively low nutrient-density when it comes to the amounts of vitamins, minerals, trace elements, antioxidants, fibre, phytochemicals, amino acids and beneficial unsaturated fatty acids per gram or per calorie.

4. An omega-3 to omega-6 fatty acid ratio that differs profoundly from that of our ancestors. Furthermore, a lower unsaturated to saturated fat ratio.

5. A high sodium content.

6. A lower content of pre- and probiotics.

7. A different impact on net acidity versus alkalinity.

8. The effects of xenohormesis on our hormones and gene expression (see *Table 1*). We are affected by external molecules and respond to them. These include xenobiotics such as mercury, dioxins, polychlorinated biphenyls (PCBs), phthalates, polybrominated diphenyl ethers and other environmental contaminants.

In short, modern foods and diets have all the required characteristics necessary to impair both brain function and general health.

TABLE 1: XENOHORMETIC SIGNALS IN FOOD

Signal	Effects	In modern man
Inflammatory messenger molecules	Inflammation, alterations in digestion, altered metabolism, alterations in brain function	Increased levels
Insulin	Changes in blood sugar levels, increased growth of various tissues	Increased levels
High levels of saturated long-chain fatty acids compared to polyunsaturated fatty acids of the omega-3 and omega-6 families and monounsaturated fatty acids	Neurological, immunological (inflammation) and metabolic responses (increased energy storage/ decreased energy expenditure) to stress signals	Increased levels
Trans fats and other damaged fatty acids	Induction of stress and injury response mechanisms, inflammation, interference with the uptake, transport and utilisation of essential fats	Increased levels
Phytochemicals such as lycopene, resveratrol, curcumin, tocopherols, isothiocyanates and catechins	Increased longevity, increased antioxidant defence capacity, improved metabolism, improved detoxification	Decreased levels

Food is more than a source of energy and nutrients – food is also information. Modern food is deprived of constituents that work like an instruction manual: telling the body how to utilise the energy and nutrients found in the foods ingested. Modern refined foods contain substances that put the body into a state of high alert – this translates into inflammation and an increased stress response.

Emerging links between brain function, diet and general health

The brain is similar to the rest of the body in that it requires a steady supply of energy and preferably not just sufficient, but optimum, amounts of macro- and micronutrients. Modern diets are rarely capable of satisfying these demands. There is a startling difference in brain function and health when providing the brain with just enough energy and nutrients to avoid frank deficiency, compared to providing ideal amounts of energy and nutrients. This obviously impacts on brain function in the short as well as long term, similar to what researchers are finding with most other diseases of civilisation.

Last but not least, the brain is sensitive to oxidative stress and inflammation (ie. when the immune system is activated in response to a perceived threat). Inflammation plays a major role in cardiovascular disease, cancer and all other modern health problems. Inflammation can be created by, as well as cause, oxidative stress, which is the equivalent of a fire out of control at the cellular and molecular level. It is now emerging that inflammation and oxidative stress play major roles in mental and neurological dysfunction and can be influenced by nutritional factors.

Mitochondria, energy and oxidative stress

An unappreciated fact in terms of diet and brain function is that neurons (nerve cells) contain large numbers of mitochondria. Mitochondria are organelles inside cells responsible for converting sugars, fats and some amino acids into useable energy. Mitochondria also create substances that are used extensively in the body's antioxidant defences and for repair, maintenance, structure and signalling. The number of mitochondria in neurons rivals that found in the heart, liver and kidneys.

The reason for this is that the central nervous system (CNS) has massive energy requirements, despite its small size, compared with the rest of the body. The CNS might use as much as half the available blood sugar and oxygen under certain circumstances, but it makes up less than two per cent of body weight in adults. There are no muscular contractions requiring energy, all signals in the brain are transmitted as electrical impulses along neurons. A very steady supply of energy is required, not only to create these impulses, but also to stop the transmission of signals.

This is of major importance for brain function. The CNS is bombarded with signals every second (eg. sensory input from eyes, ears, tactile information, taste, smell, information about blood pressure, blood sugar levels, hormone levels, oxygen levels, pulse) and has to choose what is of importance, what to act on and what to ignore. Without readily available energy, this is a difficult job. Not eating regularly, or eating food that does not release its energy and nutrients steadily and slowly, will undermine brain function.

The generation of energy in the mitochondria is equally dependent on ideal levels of nutrients. Furthermore, ideal levels of various nutrients are required to prevent the mitochondria from causing oxidative stress when they generate energy, resulting in the release of free radicals and increased cellular degeneration.

The production of serotonin, dopamine, noradrenaline and similar neurotransmitters is costly in terms of energy and requires ideal levels of numerous co-factors, such as iron, niacin, folate, vitamin B12, pyridoxine (vitamin B6), thiamine (vitamin B1), biotin, pantothenic acid (vitamin B5), selenium, vitamin C, magnesium and zinc. Nutritional status also affects how neurons (and hence the brain) perceive and act on the signals they receive.

In short, the brain has significant requirements in terms of energy supply and nutrient levels. It is rather greedy and will 'throw tantrums' when its requirements in terms of energy supply and nutrients are not met. Modern diets and lifestyles do not meet the brain's requirements. In fact, they significantly undermine brain function.

Food and the 'psychoneuroendocrine' connection

The hypothalamus in the brain is fed signals from our sensory system, our immune system, our endocrine system (as it monitors hormonal levels) and our limbic system (the part of the brain involved in learning, memory and 'attaching' emotions to events and experiences). Overload in the nervous, endocrine or immune systems will affect the other systems that are 'connected' in the hypothalamus. Modern foods are capable of causing inflammation and inducing a stress response via cytokines, cortisol and other signalling substances, and are therefore directly linked to the way the brain functions.

Cytokines are immune messengers created in response not only to infection, tissue damage or immunological processes, but also in response to:

- rapid increases in blood sugar and the subsequent increase in insulin levels
- greater concentrations of saturated fatty acids being absorbed from the digestive system
- the ingestion of trans fats
- increasing levels of inflammatory messenger molecules in foods
- ingesting foods one is allergic or intolerant to
- alterations in gut flora.

Modern foods and diets cause or contribute to all of these. Their impact on brain function can be expected to be as detrimental as continual low level stress, chronic pain that is never quite resolved, smoking and sleep deprivation.

Brain-derived neurotrophic factor

Research into brain-derived neurotrophic factor (BdNF) provides further evidence that foods and a lifestyle similar to those found in our ancestral environment are directly linked to better brain functioning. The messenger molecule BdNF plays an important role in normal neural development and encourages the growth and differentiation of neurons and synapses. The more BdNF present, the healthier the brain is. Exercise, sufficient sleep, omega-3 fatty acids, steady blood sugar levels and frequent small meals all increase BdNF levels. Smoking, stress, insufficient sleep, inflammation, imbalanced blood sugar and oxidative stress decrease BdNF levels, which in turn leads to greater brain dysfunction. Modern foods and modern lifestyles accelerate brain decay by lowering BdNF levels.

Neuroactive food constituents

Modern diets contain rapidly increasing numbers of neuroactive constituents that are capable of interfering with neurological function in the short as well as long term. Some of these are outlined here.

Refined sugar and other high-glycaemic carbohydrates

Cocaine is not the only white powder with addictive qualities affecting both body and mind that is both cheap and readily available. Refined sugar is the other one! This is a bold statement, increasingly supported by modern science. Animal studies and brain scans on humans have revealed disturbing information about the effect of refined sugar and other high-glycaemic carbohydrates. Animal studies on rats have demonstrated that:

- they can be addicted to a sweet sugar solution as fast as they can be addicted to cocaine and nicotine
- they can be weaned off cocaine and nicotine by providing enough refined sugar
- long-term changes in brain structure, function, chemistry and gene expression are very similar – whether the rats were addicted to cocaine, nicotine or sugar.

For ethical reasons, there are no studies comparing the neurological affects of consuming refined sugar and other rapidly digested and very sweet carbohydrates versus cocaine, nicotine, cannabis or other mood-altering substances in humans. Yet we have a very clear idea of how the brain responds to addictive substances whether legal (nicotine) or illegal (cannabis, cocaine, MDMA, amphetamine), both in the short and long term. PET and SPECT scans have now been performed on human subjects after the ingestion of refined sugar, among other foods. The observed effects on brain function were disturbingly close to what would be expected after snorting a line of cocaine or having a nicotine fix. In plain language: refined sugar and highly refined carbohydrates have effects very similar to both legal and illegal drugs. They interfere with brain function and are addictive.

Gluten and casein

Gluten is found in wheat, rye, barley and to some extent in oats and in 'ancient' wheat varieties such as spelt, emmer and kamut. If gluten is not completely broken down during digestion, opioid peptides called gluteomorphins can be created. The latter part of the name, '-morphins', says it all. These substances are structurally and functionally related to morphine, heroin and opium and may be released during the digestion of gluten, if not broken down completely. These are absorbed and cross the blood–brain barrier where they interfere with signalling in the brain.

The dairy protein casein, which, incidentally, is found in greater concentrations in milk from the cattle predominantly used in modern animal husbandry, also yields opioids known as casomorphins.

These neuroactive substances appear to play a role in autism, Asperger's syndrome and less severe behavioural, learning and developmental disorders such as ADHD and dyslexia. They are found at very elevated levels in the urine of many individuals with such disorders when they consume glutenous grains and dairy products, but not in people without such disorders. The levels of food-derived opioids fall when glutenous grains and dairy products are removed from the diet of people with such disorders and are often followed by improvement if dairy products and gluten are strictly avoided. If given to rats, gluteomorphins and casomorphins induce abnormal behaviour similar to that which characterises developmental, learning and behavioural disorders. Taking children off gluten and dairy products should preferably be done in collaboration with a specialist. Be aware that once removed, re-introduction of even tiny amounts can cause strong reactions.

Additives and allergies

The old-fashioned, but entrenched, view that allergies and additives cannot play a role in hyperactivity and similar disorders is puzzling. Histamine is released when we are exposed to foods and food constituents that we do not tolerate, such as artificial colours. As histamine is also an excitatory neurotransmitter, it has a general stimulating effect on brain function and activity. Excessive levels of histamine lead to excess brain activity and alterations in behaviour, thinking and emotions. Furthermore, histamine levels in the brain play a role in activating the stress response. The more histamine, the greater the stress response. Stress also interferes with learning, emotions, memory and other aspects of brain function.

Conclusion

While much more research on the extent to which modern foods are incompatible with our genetic inheritance is desirable, there is enough scientific evidence already to show that our modern diet and lifestyle is damaging our physical and mental health. Implementing a diet that shares many of the characteristics of the diets that our ancestors consumed is the way forward if we want to achieve optimum health and reverse the epidemic of degenerative disease and mental ill health. The main characteristics of such a diet are as follows.

1. No added or refined sugar. Sweetness must come from real food such as fruits and berries, as well as spices.

2. No refined grains at all and no glutenous grains for some. Eat whole grains and true whole-grain products, but not to the extent that they decrease vegetable and fruit intake below 600 g per day for adults and teenagers.

3. Eat the right fats rather than no fat. The type and quality of fat is crucial. Increase the intake of omega-3 fatty acids, unrefined fats from crops (nuts, seeds, unrefined oils) and fats from animal products that are naturally lean and have a high omega-3 fatty acid content and a low saturated to unsaturated fat ratio. Trans fats, refined fats and the fats found in animal products from grain-fed livestock should be avoided.

4. Dairy products are not absolutely essential and are a problem for some people, who do better leaving them out of their diet entirely. Any dairy products consumed, provided one can tolerate them, should be organic, unsweetened and preferably fermented (eg. plain, live yoghurt, kefir).

5. A higher nutrient density is achieved by eating organic and unrefined foods. Extra supplementation with multivitamins, essential fatty acids, probiotics and single nutrients might also be necessary to compensate for hampered digestion, decreased utilisation and increased demands.

It is important to remember that food literally speaks to your body and that your body will answer back. Speak in a loving tone (ie. eat 'real' food your body can actually 'understand') and your body will respond in kind. Glycaemic overload, trans fats and other damaged fatty acids, excess long-chain saturated fats, foreign chemicals, stress signals in animal products due to aggressive farming and livestock production, low nutrient density due to intensive farming and rearing methods – all these are the nutritional equivalent of subjecting your body to offensive language, and your body and brain will respond in kind.

Further information

Several co-authors will cover some of the topics mentioned here in more depth. Other sources of information about the various aspects of modern foods that are incompatible with our genetic heritage can be found on the following websites [all accessed May 2008].

- Loren Cordain, PhD: www.thepaleodiet.com
- Professor Jennifer Brand-Miller, Sydney University: www.glycemicindex.com
- Dr David Ludwig, Boston Children's Hospital: www.endingthefoodfight.com
- Defeat Autism Now! (DAN!): www.defeatautismnow.com
- Food and Brain Research: www.fabresearch.org
- The World's Healthiest Food: www.whfoods.com

Reference

Cordain L, Eaton SB, Sebastian A, Mann N, Lindeberg S, Watkins BA, O'Keefe JH and Brand-Miller J (2005) Origins and evolution of the Western diet: health implications for the 21st century. *The American Journal of Clinical Nutrition* **81** (2) 341–354.

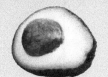

Chapter 2
Mental health and mineral depletion
DR DAVID THOMAS DC

I was once told a story about a group of blind people who were asked to describe an elephant; each duly felt the part that they were closest to and gave a remarkably accurate description. This simple analogy illustrates the many different individual research topics there have been, and that are currently being examined, in the name of nutritional research. There is a danger of losing sight of the whole 'nutrition' picture. My specific contribution relates to the research work conducted on the historical loss of minerals in our foods (Thomas, 2003; Thomas, 2007). In this article we shall consider how this circumstance relates to the myth of the 'healthy, balanced diet' and the relevance of this link to physical and mental health.

Due to my geological background, my personal preference concerning guidance to patients regarding supplementing dietary regimes has always been towards minerals and trace elements. My initial use of mineral supplementation was using Blackmore's mineral celloid therapy, and I was later introduced to a liquid trace element product called Beres Drops Plus. This product was developed by a Hungarian Biochemist, Dr Beres, who, in the 1960s, was given the research task by the Hungarian government of ascertaining why there had been successive potato crop failures in a certain part of Hungary. Dr Beres' conclusions were what many gardeners could have told him – the health of the crop depended on the health of the soil. His research demonstrated that there were a number of what he considered to be essential trace elements missing in the soil. When these were replaced, healthy crops were grown.

As a result of these insights, Dr Beres turned his attention to human diseases using the same concept: that human disease conditions relate to specific or multiple trace element deficiencies. His contention was that eventually the body's ability to adapt, compensate and adjust to continued trace element deficiency is exceeded, and disease symptoms relating to the individual genetic make-up of the person concerned will manifest. He formulated the Beres Drops Plus, which contains 17 trace elements 'blended' together with organic carrier molecules. This product is now classified as a drug in Hungary, under the category of 'roborant'. It is used specifically as an adjunct in chemotherapy and radiotherapy to minimise the side effects of these therapies.

In 1999 I was introduced to American Herbalist Paul Bergner who had observed that the successful protocol he had used with his patients over a 20-year period – a wholefood diet together with appropriate herbal tinctures – had become less effective during the past 10 years. As the tinctures had not changed, he decided to research the 'wholefood'. He discovered a dramatic decrease in many of the minerals and trace elements present in the vegetables, fruit and meats available to the American public at the time of his research, in comparison to 20 to 30 years previously (Bergner, 1997). A subsequent report by Halweil describes the loss of nutrient levels in the US food supply due to the pursuit of high yields (Halweil, 2007).

I decided to conduct similar research projects on the foods available to us in the UK. *Table 1* represents a weighted average summary of the mineral and trace element changes that have taken place for 72 foods. These can be traced through the six editions of McCance and Widdowson's *The Composition of Foods* (Food Standards Agency) between 1940 and 1991 for fruit and vegetables, and between 1940/1960 and 2002 for meat and meat products, cheeses and dairy products. For specifics regarding the foods within the categories mentioned and the details of individual losses, I would refer the reader to my original texts (Thomas, 2003; 2007). Collectively, there has been an average 19% loss in magnesium, a 29% loss in calcium, a 37% loss in iron and a really alarming 62% loss in copper – iron and copper being the only trace elements analysed in 1940.

TABLE 1: HISTORICAL ESSENTIAL MINERAL DEPLETION CHANGES IN FIVE CATEGORIES OF FOOD PRODUCTS

	1940–1991 Vegetables (n = 28)	1940–1991 Fruit (n = 17)	1940–2002 Meat (n = 14)	1940–2002 Cheeses (n = 9)	1940–2002 Dairy (n = 4)	Weighted average (n = 72)
Sodium	-49%	-29%	-24%	-9%	-47%	-34%
Potassium	-16%	-19%	-9%	-19%	-7%	-15%
Phosphorus	9%	2%	-21%	-8%	34%	1%
Magnesium	-24%	-16%	-15%	-26%	-1%	-19%
Calcium	-46%	-16%	-29%	-15%	4%	-29%
Iron	-27%	-24%	-50%	-53%	-83%	-37%
Copper	-76%	-20%	-55%	-91%	-97%	-62%

Table 2 shows the loss of minerals (including zinc) in seven vegetables that were analysed by McCance and Widdowson, subsequent to 1940, over the 13-year period 1978 to 1991. Unfortunately, only seven vegetables could be traced and the results are again disconcerting.

TABLE 2: MINERAL CHANGES IN VEGETABLES BETWEEN 1978 AND 1991

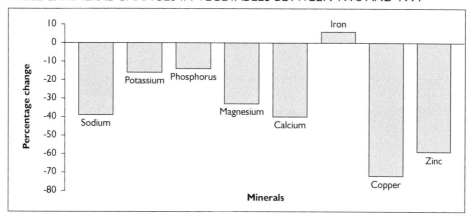

To try and put the significance of these findings into perspective, let's consider the approximate recommended daily allowances (RDAs) for magnesium (300 mg), zinc (10 mg) and chromium (100 mcg), remembering that in the view of many nutritionists, the RDAs are considered the absolute minimums before deficiency disease conditions begin to manifest. How much is this actually per day? Consider that just over half a teaspoon represents your magnesium quota; a 50th of a teaspoon is the requirement for zinc; while a 500th of a teaspoon is all that is required for chromium. In relationship to the amount of food we eat each day, these are minuscule amounts.

Magnesium-rich foods include: green leafy vegetables; meats; wholegrains; milk; nuts and seeds, such as sunflower and pumpkin.

Zinc-rich foods include: oysters; lamb; pecan nuts; peas; haddock; potatoes; egg-yolk; peanuts; sardines; tuna; lentils.

Chromium-rich foods include: organ meats; mushrooms; broccoli; oysters.

Although broccoli is rich in minerals, 100 g only contains 13 mg of magnesium (4.3% of RDA) and 0.4 mg of zinc (4% of RDA). In other words, you would have to eat 2.5 kg of broccoli per day to satisfy the RDA. It gets worse: the micronutrients in foods are present in many different forms and some are more readily assimilated than others. Iron from animal tissues (haem) has greater bioavailability than iron present in vegetables. So, although analytically certain foods may be rich in certain minerals (eg. iron in spinach), the amount assimilated is significantly less than is actually in the food. In addition, there are complex synergistic inter-relationships that exist between these various essential micronutrients. Too much zinc, for instance, will interfere with copper metabolism.

Finally, it is not just what you eat, it is also what your body is able to absorb from what you eat. If the gastrointestinal tract has been compromised, this will make an optimum digestive process less likely. Another major culprit associated with poor absorption is mental and emotional stress. The biodiversity within the human race also plays an important role – because of inherent genetic-constitutional traits, the same deficiency will manifest itself in different ways in different individuals.

Magnesium and zinc both play vital neurological roles, and deficiency symptoms include: sensitivity to noise; nervousness; irritability; mental depression; confusion; twitching; trembling; apprehension; insomnia; muscle weakness; ADHD; anorexia nervosa; bulimia nervosa; amnesia; apathy; depression; irritability; lethargy; mental retardation; paranoia.

Chromium deficiency is associated with: depression; insulin resistance; mood swings.

These days it is very difficult to obtain a 'healthy, balanced diet'. Given this, and the fact that micronutrient deficiency can be an integral and fundamental component of all disease conditions, does it not make sense in a therapeutic situation to give people the choice of sound dietary guidance and appropriate supplementation (and observe how they progress), prior to dispensing pharmaceutical and psychopharmacological drugs? The very ingestion of the latter may not only further deplete body reserves of essential micronutrients, but detrimentally interfere with their bioavailability.

In my initial paper I listed some of the physical, mental and emotional conditions that are influenced by mineral and trace element deficiencies (Thomas, 2003). In my second paper I was able to reference 214 peer-reviewed research papers written between 1923 and 2003 that correlate specific mental illnesses with specific mineral and trace element deficiencies or imbalances (Thomas, 2007). **Table 3** represents a summary of these papers.

TABLE 3: MENTAL ILLNESSES CORRELATED WITH MINERAL AND TRACE ELEMENT DEFICIENCIES OR IMBALANCES

	Chromium	Copper	Iron	Iodine	Potassium	Magnesium	Molybdenum	Phosphorus	Selenium	Vanadium	Zinc
ADHD		X				X		X			X
Anxiety					X	X		X	X		
Aggression			X		X						X
Bipolar disorder			X	X	X	X	X			X	
Depression	X	X	X	X	X	X			X	X	X
PMS		X	X			X					X
Schizophrenia		X	X	X		X			X		

As individuals, and as a society as a whole, we are aware that eating is a fundamental requirement for life and that what we eat is relevant to our health. Awareness that food can affect health has been part of our national psyche from as long ago as the early 17th century, when it was realised that scurvy was caused by a lack of fresh fruit and vegetables. Yet, from an 'establishment' perspective, the essential role of micronutrients (eg. minerals, trace elements, vitamins, essential fatty acids, phytonutrients, digestive enzymes, probiotics) is cursory at best and usually ignored. The best guidance is to 'eat a healthy, balanced diet'. This is a very difficult directive when the presence of micronutrients is diminishing and the modern diet favours meals high in proteins, carbohydrates and saturated fats, colourings, flavourings and preservatives.

Warnings, research and relevant information have existed since the 1930s, written by many esteemed men and women working as pioneers in the fields of nutrition and health, including Sir Robert McCarrison (1936; 1937), Surgeon Captain TL Cleave RN (1977), Weston Price (1945), Linus Pauling (1970) and Trowell, Burkitt and Heaton (1986) among many others. Perhaps to emphasise the fundamental role that micronutrients play in our physical and psychological well-being (and their global relevance to health), in March 2006 the UN acknowledged a 'new' kind of malnutrition. Catherine Bertini (2006), Chairperson of the UN Standing Committee on Nutrition, said:

> 'The overweight are just as malnourished as the starving, and nutritional programs in poor countries need to target rising obesity alongside hunger.'

She also suggested that we need a new definition of malnutrition because food availability is not really the issue – the *quality* of food is the problem. A new type of malnutrition has been recognised that can be categorised as multiple micronutrient depletion and has been termed 'type B malnutrition'.

To re-emphasise this point, despite a huge amount of research evidence and past and current campaigning by many organisations – including The McCarrison Society, Foresight, the Alliance for Natural Health, Sustain and the Hyperactive Children's Support Group – very little heed is given to their research results or 'real life' experiences. Recently, Lauridsen *et al* (2006) found that rats fed on organic food were less fat, slept better and had stronger immune systems than rats fed on conventionally grown produce. Given the enormous knowledge base on the significance of good nutrition in relationship to good health, these findings are common sense. Is it worthwhile to continue to prove the obvious?

Examples of ongoing research needed in this field are currently being promoted by The Good Gardeners Association's *Moving Beyond Organic* project and the Tablehurst Farm initiative *Learning on the Land* (www.tablehurstandplawhatch.co.uk). The aim of *Moving Beyond Organic* is to develop research methods that link the well-being of the micro life of a soil to an increase in the food's nutritional qualities. Working in partnership, this experimental research work is being developed in a garden called GREEN (Gardens for Research Experimental Education and Nutrition) (Good Gardeners Association, 2006). Using quantitative and qualitative methods, the flow of minerals, trace minerals and other nutrients, as well as the 'life force' from soil to plant are being tracked. The objective is to learn how these processes are affected by the method of cultivation used and the subsequent effect that this has on the soil food-web.

Preliminary findings suggest that to grow nutritious food, knowledge of soil biology is far more useful than soil chemistry. When plants are encouraged to form symbiotic relationships with beneficial soil microbes, it appears to increase the transfer of essential nutrients from soil to plant. To date, this research has produced potatoes and leeks with substantial increases in calcium, magnesium and iron that far exceed any of the data from 1940. As the methodology develops, more tests are being added (the latest being antioxidants), which again show variations depending on soil health. This research project should be applauded – and publicly funded.

The *Learning on the Land* initiative recognises the historical separation that has taken place between individuals (particularly children) and where their food originates. It seeks, by inviting school children to live within a working farm environment, to reassert the connection that arable and pastoral foods have on soil preparation, cultivation and production, and then the role that cooking and community sharing of the produce has on their social life.

As the many research references used indicate, the quality of the food and drink we consume does make a difference to our physical, mental and emotional health. The impact of the decline in micronutrients in modern foods compared with foods available 70 years ago is exacerbated by two further problems:

■ a substantial proportion of the population consume few or no fresh vegetables at all

■ 'modern' foods contain various other components that come as 'part of the package', namely residual herbicides, pesticides, fungicides and the ubiquitous additives of processed, convenience foods, eg. colourings, flavourings, preservatives (while some of these have been individually tested for short-term safety, no one knows what their interactions might be or their cumulative effects on the body over a lifetime).

The question then arises as to what is to be done about this potentially catastrophic state of affairs. During the Second World War the UK government required that, because diets might be inadequate due to rationing, all children should receive cod liver oil and orange juice. Sixty years on, despite the historical 'official' introduction of 'fortified foods' we find that we are in a situation where the nation, as a whole, is overfed but malnourished. Supplementation and fortification can certainly play a role and this is a subject for research and debate in its own right (Mejia, 1994; Fletcher *et al*, 2004).

REASONS FOR THE REDUCTION IN THE MINERAL CONTENT OF FOOD OVER TIME

- Favouring varieties of crops and animal breeds for their presentation rather than nutritional quality.

- Increased use of NPK fertilisers free of trace elements.

- Inevitable soil depletion of essential minerals through continuous crop growing, contributed to by the overuse of NPK fertilisers with consequent damage to endomycorrhizal fungi that help liberate essential minerals from the soil (Ward et al, 2001).

- Inherent soil deficiencies of essential minerals due to parent bedrock material, the amount of organic matter present, the ionic potential of differing trace elements, the degree of soil oxidisation and soil pH (Thorvaldsson, 2005).

- Increased transport distances, storage times and storage methods for 'fresh' produce.

FACTORS CONTRIBUTING TO MINERAL DEPLETION IN THE POPULATION

- Increased lifestyle stresses: mental, physical and emotional.

- Increased use of stimulants: coffee, tea, tobacco, alcohol and recreational drugs.

- Increased use of medication.

- Dietary trends towards cheaper, more refined, quicker, convenience foods and drinks, which are high in proteins, saturated fats and refined carbohydrates but very low in micronutrients.

- Polluted air and water supplies.

- Sunlight deprivation and quality (due to ozone depletion).

The form that supplementation takes is vital, as if it is too 'crude', the supplement is likely to leave the body in exactly the manner it went in. Also, given that it is possible to upset the balance between specific minerals/trace elements, I would suggest that if daily supplementation is considered, it should be derived from a naturally-occurring sea/food source (chlorella, kelp, spirulina, sea water concentrates, cod liver oil, brewers yeast, fruit concentrates).

Supplementation may well prove to be a constructive short to medium-term solution but only if, at the same time, we actively encourage lifestyle changes from an early age. These should include:

- exercising
- healthier eating and drinking habits
- paying specific attention to advertising and the availability and presentation of junk food in schools, hospitals, penal institutions and public places.

There is a desperate need for the conventional farming and food and drink industries to become more aware of their role in this scenario and realise that they have an ever-growing responsibility to their customers to provide good-quality, nourishing, non-toxic products. More 'holistic' and local projects, such as those being developed by GREEN and *Learning on the Land* should be encouraged and publicly funded. Fortunately, there has been an interesting, relatively recent, positive development: a significant and growing trend towards nutritional awareness. This is demonstrated by the buying of locally grown and organic produce and a greater interest in food preparation, world cuisine and animal husbandry – a powerful force, and one that is likely to bring about significant changes in the food industry.

Already, this consumer-driven change has resulted in alterations in food labelling, as well as greater availability of organically and bio-dynamically grown foods. We have recently experienced a resistant, but gradual, decline in the addition of additives to foods in the food and drink industries, especially artificial colours and preservatives, sugar, salt and trans fats. In addition, the cooking of foods has been given far greater emphasis both through media attention nationally and via specific informative sites.

To return to my initial comments about the elephant: this article is not 'just' about the loss of micronutrients in our food over historical time and the proven relationship of micronutrients to physiological and psychological health, it is about becoming more aware of the importance and significance of those bountiful resources, which are ultimately the providers of our 'nourishment' – the land and the sea. In so doing, it should be possible to consciously re-assert our relationship with our environment and thereby appreciate the appropriate stewardship that is necessary to care correctly for them. A true respect of these resources and the fundamental role that nutrition plays in our lives would lead us – individually and collectively – to procure, prepare, cook, present and celebrate our food in a far more considered and conscious manner than is currently evident.

HOW TO MAXIMISE YOUR MINERALS*

- Optimise every link in the chain from soil to plate by raising healthy soils, finding the best ingredients and doing the minimum to them.

- The fresher, the better – so buy local and seasonal. Look for local farmers who use compost, crop rotation and minimal digging. If you want to guarantee the health of the soil, look for the Demeter certification (biodynamic symbol).

- Try and increase the number of times you shop per week. Explore farmers' markets, farm gate shops and organic box delivery schemes (supermarket produce is likely to have clocked up food miles, storage time and chemical storage tricks).

- Choose a variety of different foods to maximise nutrient intake.

- The more colourful the produce, the higher their mineral and antioxidant levels.

- Scrub fruit and vegetables rather than peeling them, as most of the nutrients hide just under the skin.

- Cook with minimum water, heat and time. Keep the vegetable water for soup, or drink it.

- Steam or stir fry rather than deep fry, grill, char or roast.

- Store fresh produce in cool, dark places. Freeze leftovers or extra portions as soon as possible.

- Avoid foods that have been refined, processed, tinned and packaged for convenience whenever possible.

* With thanks to Jane Lorimer; see: www.janelorimerforhealth.co.uk

References

Bergner P (1997) *The Healing Power of Minerals.* Rocklin, CA: Prima Health.

Bertini C (2006) *Report of the Standing Committee on Nutrition at its 33rd Session.* Hosted by the World Health Organization, at the Geneva International Conference Centre, Geneva, Switzerland 13–17 March 2006. Available at: www.unsystem.org/SCN/Publications/AnnualMeeting/SCN33/FINAL%20REPORT%2033rd%20SESSION.pdf [accessed 28/04/08].

Cleve TL (1977) Over-consumption. Now the most dangerous cause of disease in Westernised countries. *Public Health: The Journal of the Society of Community Medicine* **91** (3) 127–123.

Fletcher RJ, Bell IP and Lambert JP (2004) Public health aspects of food fortification: a question of balance. *Proceedings of the Nutritional Society* **63** (4) 605–614.

Food Standards Agency (1940–2002) *McCance and Widdowson's The Composition of Foods* (various editions). London: Royal Society of Chemistry.

Good Gardeners Association (2006) GREEN data from *The Good Gardeners Association News Journal* **159**; **160**; **161**; **162**.

Halweil B (2007) *Still No Free Lunch: Nutrient levels in US food supply eroded by pursuit of high yields.* Critical issue report for The Organic Center. Available at: www.organic-center.org/reportfiles/Yield_Nutrient_Density_Final.pdf [accessed 28/04/08].

Lauridsen C, Jørgensen H, Halekoh U, Porskjær Christensen L and Brandt K (2006) Organic diet enhanced the health of rats. Website: *Danish Research Centre for Organic Food and Farming.* Available at: www.darcof.dk/research/health.html [accessed 28/04/08].

McCarrison R (1936) Nutrition in health and disease. *British Medical Journal* **2** 611–615.

McCarrison R (1937) Nutritional needs in pregnancy. *British Medical Journal* **2** 256–257.

Mejia LA (1994) Fortification of foods: historical development and current practices. *Food and Nutrition Bulletin* **15** (4) 278–281.

Pauling L (1970) Evolution and the need for ascorbic acid. *Proceedings of the National Academy of Sciences* **67** (4).

Price W (1945) *Nutrition and Physical Degeneration.* New Canaan, CT: Keats Publishing.

Thomas DE (2003) A study of the mineral depletion of foods available to us as a nation over the period 1940 to 1991. *Nutrition and Health* **17** (2) 85–115.

Thomas DE (2007) The mineral depletion of foods available to us as a nation over the period 1940 to 2002. *Nutrition and Health* **19** 21–55.

Thorvaldsson G (2005) *Essential Trace Elements for Plants, Animals and Humans.* NJF Seminar 370 convened by Agricultural University of Iceland. Available at: www.hvanneyri.is/landbunadur/wglbhi.nsf/Attachment/LBHI-rit-3/$file/LBHI-rit-3.pdf [accessed 28/04/08].

Trowell N, Burkitt D and Heaton K (1986) *Dietary Fibre, Fibre-depleted Foods and Disease.* London: Academic Press.

Ward N, Stead K and Reeves J (2001) Impact of endomycorrhizal fungi on plant trace element uptake and nutrition. *The Nutrition Practitioner* **3** (2) 30–31.

Chapter 3
The influence of chemical additives on children's behaviour
DR BRIAN MCDONOGH

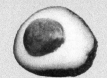

Have you, like me, ever wondered why there are so many additives in foods (in particular sweets), drinks and medicines?

What are food additives?
Food additives are substances deliberately added to food by the manufacturer for one or more of the following reasons:

- in order to facilitate processing
- to improve the appearance, texture and/or flavour
- to retain the quality or nutritional value (bear in mind that synthetic additives have no nutritional value of their own).

The use of chemical additives has been borne out of our knowledge and experience of the properties of familiar kitchen ingredients. For example, sodium bicarbonate (raising agent, browning agent and preservative), pectin (gelling agent), acetic acid (preservative), egg-yolk (emulsifier), lemon juice (antioxidant and preservative), gluten (binding agent) and sugar (sweetener and preservative).

The European Food Safety Authority is the body responsible for all food safety matters in the EU. It allocates an 'E' number to food additives (synthetic or natural) that have been cleared after safety testing and evaluation. This is to make them systematically identifiable, for example:

- E100–E199: colours
- E200–E299: preservatives
- E300–E399: antioxidants
- E400 plus: others.

EU law states that food additives are only allowed if they present no hazard to health at the level used in food and if a *reasonable need* for the additive can be demonstrated. In the UK it is the Food Standards Agency (FSA) that enforces the EU regulations.

At the outset I would like to highlight that some food additives are absolutely necessary in processed foods. Without them, many products could not be kept in a satisfactory state during storage, packaging, transport and shelf-life. In other words, food additives play an essential role in the modern world to assure the adequate supply of quality food.

However, the questions we should be asking are as follows.
1. Are all of the many additives found in some foods, drinks and medicines necessary?
2. Are they really completely safe?
3. Could, and should, some synthetic additives be replaced by natural ones, even if they are more expensive to isolate and produce?
4. What lessons can be learned and implemented?

Why are additives necessary?

The main categories of food additives listed here go some way to explain why they are added.

Preservatives

To prevent food going off quickly, for example, sulphur dioxide in wine and beer, calcium propionate in bread and sodium nitrite in processed meats. Benzoic acid and sodium benzoate are used as preservatives in a wide range of foods, drinks and medicines.

Antioxidants

To prevent oxidation (rancidity). All foodstuffs, especially fats and oils, are vulnerable to oxidation. Examples are the addition of tocopherols to fat for making cakes and ascorbyl palmitate to margarine. The most common synthetic antioxidants are butylated hydroxyanisole (BHA) and butylated hydroxytoluene (BHT).

Gelling, thickening and stabilising

These influence texture and consistency. They are gums such as pectins in jam and locust bean gum in ice cream. Gums are polysaccharides, which have an affinity for water, resulting in a gel rather than a solution.

Emulsifiers

To keep fats/oils dispersed in water, for example, lecithin in chocolate, mono- and di-glycerides in ice cream and alginates (from seaweed) in many products. Milk is the classic emulsion. Bread goes stale very quickly without emulsifiers being added.

Flavouring

To impart flavour, for example, monosodium glutamate in some potato crisps, stocks, tenderising agents and packet sauces and soups.

Colours

To replace colour lost in processing and to impart colour, for example, carotenes in cheese and margarine and carmoisine in soft drinks. Synthetic colours are used instead of the natural ones because the extraction of natural colours is often neither practical nor economical. The first additive colours were synthetic dyes made mainly from coal tar (these are now called azo dyes). The use of artificial colours merely to impart colour is not essential, but is intended to make the foodstuff more visually appealing. Azo dyes are the largest group of certified colourants. They are characterised by the presence of one or more azo (double nitrogen) bonds (-N=N-). They are permitted in any food except raw or processed meat, fish, fruit, vegetables, white bread, tea, coffee and milk (Coultate, 1984).

Sweeteners

To provide sweetness without calories or simply to replace sugar, eg. the intense sweeteners (eg. aspartame, acesulfame K, saccharin, sucralose, alitame) and bulk sweeteners (eg. xylitol, lactitol, maltitol). Natural sweeteners are sugar and honey.

Acids

To impart sharpness of flavour, for example, phosphoric acid in cola drinks. Acids can also have preservative and antioxidant effects, such as citric acid from lemons, malic acid in apples and tartaric acid in grapes. In quantity, phosphoric and citric acids can cause tooth decay. Phosphoric acid can also reduce magnesium levels (Johnson, 2001).

There is no essential difference in the chemical structure of synthetic (artificial) versus natural additives. Many synthetic additives are simply chemical copies of the natural equivalent, for example, citric acid and sodium benzoate. Yet, many are totally foreign to living organisms, such as the azo dye colourants and phosphoric acid.

The argument posed by the Food Additives and Ingredients Association (FAIA) is that, given the fact that there are so many additives in processed foods, sweets and drinks today, it is inevitable that some individuals will be intolerant to some of them. One would gather from this that they believe that adverse reactions are simply random and, therefore, that the use of so many food additives is justified. Whatever the standpoint, when increasing suspicion is placed at the door of particular additives, as we shall see from the research, there is obviously more to the problem than purely random effects.

It is worth noting that there are certain characteristics common to a subgroup of people sensitive to food additives (Joneja, 1998; 2001):

- a history of asthma or allergic rhinitis (atopic diseases)
- a history or family history of aspirin sensitivity
- a history or family history of migraine.

Do any additives cause harm?

It is chiefly the azo dye colours, flavourants, such as monosodium glutamate, preservatives, such as the sodium benzoate family and some strong sweeteners that have focused the attention of practitioners dealing with various illnesses such as attention deficit hyperactivity disorder (ADHD), asthma and eczema.

ADHD is a condition mainly affecting children and is characterised by inattention (lack of concentration), hyperactivity and impulsivity – leading to academic and social impairment.

We will look at the evidence that additives may cause, or aggravate, ADHD. There have been reports from many practitioners over many decades that the behaviour of children with this diagnosis can improve significantly when certain artificial additives are excluded. Unfortunately, many of these have been reported as case studies; modern science prefers double-blind, placebo-controlled studies, which are very difficult to design properly when attempting to assess food-related issues. As a result, many such trials have been flawed in one way or another. Excellent overall discussion of these trials is given by Professor Erik Millstone (1997).

In the UK the overall incidence of acute adverse reactions in all children to food additives lies somewhere between 1% and 20% (Millstone, 1997). However, the incidence in children with ADHD has been reported to be as high as 80% (Egger *et al*, 1985; Feingold, 1975; Ward *et al*, 1990; Conners *et al*, 1976).

Numerous research projects have verified that eliminating exposure to additives can improve the mental and behavioural functioning of children with ADHD. In 1975, Dr Benjamin Feingold, a Paediatrician and Allergist, found that up to half of children with ADHD returned to normal behaviour when primarily synthetic colourants and flavouring agents were removed from their diets (Feingold, 1975).

In 1976 Dr Keith Conners and colleagues did a controlled study on 15 children with ADHD, thinking that they would disprove Feingold's findings. Much to their surprise, they reported results that supported Feingold's findings (Conners *et al*, 1976).

Egger and colleagues (1985) reported that colourants (eg. tartrazine) and preservatives (eg. benzoates) were the commonest substances that provoked abnormal behaviour in their double-blind, placebo-controlled, cross-over trial using a low-antigenic diet in 76 cases of ADHD.

Kaplan and colleagues (1989) applied a random-allocation design trial and found that behaviour ratings of children with ADHD were better during a period of treatment with an exclusion diet than during a period on a comparison diet. The test diet excluded all food additives (including artificial colours, preservatives and flavourants) as well as food and drinks containing chocolate or caffeine.

More recently, the Food Commission (2002) reported a definite link between food additives and behaviour after studying their effects in 277 three-year-old children from the Isle of Wight. Some azo dyes (E102, E110, E122, E124) and sodium benzoate preservatives were used in the study. According to parental feedback, removal of these additives brought about a substantial improvement in hyperactive symptoms. A well-designed follow-up trial in Southampton, published in 2007 (McCann *et al*), found strong support for the case that food additives exacerbate hyperactive behaviour in children and that this can occur within one hour of consumption. The Food Standards Agency (FSA) immediately revised their advice on azo dyes, stating that children showing signs of hyperactivity may benefit from avoiding them. They did not, however, extend their advice for all children to avoid these colourants and neither did they recommend that the food industry ban their use.

The behavioural response to tartrazine is dose-dependent. Rowe and Rowe (1994) studied the effects of tartrazine on 200 ADHD children after a six-week period with no synthetic colouring. One of six dose levels of tartrazine (1 mg, 2 mg, 5 mg, 10 mg, 20 mg, 50 mg) or a placebo was administered randomly each morning. Parents of 150 children (75% cases) reported an improvement in behaviour in the withdrawal phase, but deterioration once the tartrazine was reintroduced. Symptoms included irritability, sleep disturbances, restlessness, aggression and reduced attention span. Doses over 10 mg per day produced effects for longer than 24 hours.

In a 21-day, double-blind, placebo-controlled, repeated-measures study (each child used as their own control) by the same authors, 19 of 23 suspected reactors did indeed react to tartrazine, as opposed to only two out of 20 controls. Of further interest is that all the children that reacted to tartrazine had family histories of atopic disease, such as asthma, eczema and rhinitis (Rowe and Rowe, 1994). It appears that both foods and artificial colourants are more likely to affect children from 'atopic' families.

Swanson and Kinsbourne (1980) reported that food dyes impaired the performance of hyperactive children on a laboratory learning test. Giving these additives to ADHD children increased the number of mistakes they made in a learning test, but had no effect on children who did not have ADHD. A placebo had no effect (Ward *et al*, 1990).

In the study done by Ward and colleagues (1990), a professional psychologist observed the behaviour of children over the 120-minute period after being given tartrazine and observed that after only 30 minutes:

- 18 were overactive
- 16 were aggressive
- 4 became violent
- 2 developed poor speech
- 12 developed poor co-ordination
- 8 developed asthma and/or eczema
- no behavioural problems were reported in the control group.

What other harmful effects can azo dyes have?

Concern has been growing over the inclusion of azo dyes in food as they have an effect on the following.

Serum mineral depletion (zinc, magnesium) (Ward *et al*, 1990)

Tartrazine has been shown to *reduce serum levels of zinc* (and other minerals) and amaranth can reduce magnesium levels. Tartrazine and sunset yellow have been shown to *increase urinary excretion* of zinc.

Effects of additives in an important study done by Ward and colleagues (1990) were as follows.

- **Tartrazine (E102):** 23 children with ADHD were given 50 mg tartrazine and their zinc levels (blood and urine) and behaviour were monitored for 120 minutes. After only 30 minutes, their serum zinc levels were statistically significantly lower and urinary output of zinc increased. Ward states that children with ADHD are not only low in zinc status, but seem to lose further zinc after the consumption of tartrazine. The control group of 15 children without ADHD showed stable zinc levels, normal urinary output of zinc and no behavioural changes. Low zinc status may secondarily cause reduced levels of fatty acids in children with ADHD.

- **Sunset yellow (E110):** the same dose (50 mg) of sunset yellow given to 12 children with ADHD showed the same reactions as to tartrazine, only less severe.

- **Amaranth (E123):** the same dose of amaranth (50 mg) given to 12 children with ADHD caused an increase in magnesium secretion: zinc levels were unchanged; six became overactive; eight became aggressive; one developed poor co-ordination; one developed asthma.

These findings suggest a possible chemical interaction between certain azo dyes and essential trace elements that may be linked to the aetiology of ADHD (Ward *et al*, 1990; Ward, 1997). One would question why the control groups seem unaffected by azo dyes; they may act as chelating agents, thereby reducing the absorption of trace minerals.

Digestive enzymes

Laboratory testing demonstrates that artificial food colours, such as tartrazine and sunset yellow, reduce the activity of the digestive enzymes α-amylase, pepsin and trypsin (Ward *et al*, 1990; Kroyer, 1986). This could lead to inadequate digestion, reduced nutrient availability (especially of zinc, iron and essential fatty acids) and an increased allergic/intolerance response due to antigenic loading of the gut. This means that more molecules become available to trigger the immune system. (Ward *et al*, 1990; Ward, 1997; Kroyer, 1986).

Other gastrointestinal tract effects

Low levels of trace minerals are associated with gut permeability and decreased immunity. In certain individuals, azo dyes may affect the integrity of the gut lining, leading to increased permeability and the absorption of the dye itself. Animal studies have also linked tartrazine and sunset yellow to changes in the composition of gut flora (Ward, 1997). In studies using mice, azo dyes were found to be the most genotoxic of all food additives studied, causing DNA damage in the stomach glands, colon and bladder (Sasaki *et al*, 2002).

Vitamin C levels

In 1986, Kroyer reported that the azo dyes tartrazine, cochineal red, brilliant blue and indigo carmine cause extensive breakdown of L-ascorbic acid in vitro.

Phenol sulfotransferase (PST-P)

Some azo dyes are potent inhibitors of this enzyme (Gibb *et al*, 1986). The worst offenders are carmoisine, amaranth and erythrosine. This is one of the links to migraine, which is often associated with reduced levels of PST.

Histamine

People with tartrazine sensitivity tend to have higher levels of histamine (Joneja, 1998; 2001). This means that they can get more symptoms of allergies.

Cyclo-oxygenase (COX)

This is an enzyme that causes inflammation. Azo dyes inhibit COX and, in so doing, can aggravate asthma by forcing the alternative lipoxygenase pathway in the same way that salicylates (aspirin) and other anti-inflammatory drugs do (Joneja, 1998; 2001).

Mitochondrial energy metabolism

By reducing levels of the amino acid carnitine in the body, azo dyes have been shown to reduce cellular energy production (Reyes *et al*, 1996).

Benzoates

Parents often complain about the use of sodium benzoate, an important preservative in some processed foods, because they witness behavioural changes in their children soon after they ingest it. In their double-blind, placebo-controlled, cross-over trial using a low allergenic, few-foods diet in 76 cases of ADHD, Egger and colleagues (1985) reported that preservatives, such as benzoates, commonly provoke abnormal behaviour. The mechanism may be through inhibition of the cyclo-oxygenase (COX) pathway, which would explain why aspirin-sensitive individuals, who are sensitive to COX-inhibition are particularly vulnerable to benzoate sensitivity (Jacobsen, 1991). See *Further information* for more on benzoic acid and artificial sweeteners.

What alternatives could be used?

Fortunately, food manufacturers are increasingly replacing suspect additives with ones with no known adverse effects.

- Some alternative colourants are the carotenes, curcumin, riboflavin, chlorophyll, annatto, capsanthin, xanthins, beetroot red, anthocyanins, calcium carbonate, iron oxides and hydroxides.

- Some alternative preservatives are sugar, honey, nisin (a natural antimicrobial agent derived from fermentation of *Lactococcus lactis*), acetic acid (vinegar), citric acid, sodium diacetate, calcium acetate and fumaric acid.

- Some alternative antioxidants are flavonoids (apples, onions, tomatoes, tea), L-ascorbates (vitamin C, eg. lemon juice), tocopherols (vitamin E), lecithins (egg-yolk, soya), sodium citrates, nicotinic acid, succinic acid and metatartaric acid.

What lessons can be learned?

1. The incidence of significant intolerance reactions is higher than some trials would have us believe.

2. The use of artificial colouring in food manufacture may be superfluous in that they make the product look more attractive. They are usually not essential.

3. Food additives (especially those targeted at children) that have been implicated in the provocation of problems should be far more tightly restricted. There should be more pressure on the food industry not to include suspect additives, especially where safer (not necessarily, but preferably natural) alternatives are available. Such changes should come not only from the relevant authorities, but also from consumer pressure.

4. Lessons should be learned from what other countries are doing. For example, Ponceau 4R (E124) has been banned in the US after a Federal Report concluded that it has no 'safe level', yet it is still licensed for use in the UK (*News of the World*, 2002). Other additives have been banned in various other countries.

5. If further trials are to be commissioned they should be more robustly planned so as to avoid the confounding issues so prevalent in the trials completed to date.

6. When estimating the incidence of additive intolerance, behavioural as well as atopic reactions should be considered in future trials (Millstone, 1997).

7. It is impossible to calculate the risk when using multiple combinations of additives, eg. their interactions with each other and with other compounds in the food or drink. One example is the interaction of vitamin C with sodium

benzoate to form benzene, a known cause of leukaemia and other cancers (see *Further information*).

How can we avoid food additives?

As we have seen, many food additives are simply essential to preserve and store food. It is neither practical nor advantageous to try to avoid them all.

- As far as possible buy or grow your own fresh organic produce.

- Cook and bake healthy meals at home, including bread and muffins.

- Try to avoid products that will remain 'fresh' for very long periods of time.

- Look for products (especially sweets and drinks) that do not have a long list of additives.

- Read labels! At present there is a 'buyer beware' attitude by some manufacturers. This means that the onus is on you to avoid additives you suspect may be harmful to you or your children. Don't forget to check drinks, sweets, toothpaste and medicines as well.

- Try to identify which additives are causing problems. Unfortunately, there is no blood or laboratory test that can measure intolerance to additives, so you may need the help of a nutrition practitioner.

Conclusions

Looking at the published evidence, as well as the reports from practitioners working in this field, I am convinced that the majority of children with ADHD improve (often markedly) when certain additives are excluded from their diet. It is unusual for there to be no improvement at all. Undoubtedly, such improvements are not solely due to the avoidance of additives, but also to improving the mineral status of the individual, dealing with co-existing gut problems (eg. food intolerances and overgrowth of yeast organisms) and the addition of essential fatty acids.

Looking at all of the evidence at this point, it is impossible to state that certain artificial additives, especially azo dyes, present 'no health hazard'. I am convinced that there is no longer an argument for their 'reasonable need', especially when they are deliberately targeted and marketed to unsuspecting children.

LIST OF E ADDITIVES MENTIONED IN THIS CHAPTER WITH THEIR CORRESPONDING E NUMBERS

Acesulfame K **E950**	Lecithin **E322**
Alginates **E401–E405**	Locust bean gum **E410**
Amaranth **E123**	Malic acid **E296**
Ascorbyl palmitate **E304**	Maltitol **E965**
Aspartame **E951**	Monosodium glutamate **E621**
Azo dyes **E102–133**	Pectins **E440**
Benzoates **E210–219**	Phosphoric acid **E338**
Benzoic acid **E210**	Ponceau 4R **E124**
Brilliant blue **E133**	Saccharin **E954**
Butylated hydroxyanisole (BHA) **E320**	Sodium benzoate family **E210–219**
Butylated hydroxytoluene (BHT) **E321**	Sodium benzoate **E211**
Calcium propionate **E282**	Sodium nitrite **E250**
Carmoisine **E122**	Sucralose **E955**
Carotenes **E160a**	Sulphur dioxide **E220**
Citric acid **E330**	Sunset yellow **E110**
Cochineal red **E120**	Tartaric acid **E334**
Erythrosine **E127**	Tartrazine **E102**
Indigo carmine **E132**	Tocopherols **E306**
Lactitol **E966**	Xylitol **E967**

Source: www.ukfoodguide.net

Further information

A very useful pocket guide to food additives is available from Foresight Preconception Head Office, 178 Hawthorn Road, West Bognor, West Sussex PO21 2UY; Tel: 01243 868001; Fax: 01243 868180.

Food Additives and Ingredients Association: www.faia.org.uk

DVD on aspartame called *Sweet Misery: A poisoned world:* www.mercola.com/forms/sweet_misery.htm

Article on FDA probe into benzene contamination of soft drinks: www.beveragedaily.com/news/ng.asp?id=65840

For an excellent review of the shortcomings of trials in this field as well as commentary by Professor Erik Millstone see Millstone (1997).

References

Conners CK, Goyette CH, Southwick DA, Lees JM and Andrulonis PA (1976) Food additives and hyperkinesis. A double-blind experiment. *Pediatrics* **58** (2) 154–166.

Coultate TP (1984) *Food, the Chemistry of its Components.* London: Royal Society of Chemistry.

Egger J, Carter CM, Graham PJ, Gumley D and Soothill JF (1985) Controlled trial of oligoantigenic treatment in the hyperkinetic syndrome. *The Lancet* **1** (8428) 540–545.

Feingold BF (1975) Hyperkinesis and learning disabilities linked to artificial food flavors and colors. *American Journal of Nursing* **75** 797–803.

Food Commission (2002) Additives do cause temper tantrums. *The Food Magazine* **59**.

Gibb C, Glover V and Sandler M (1986) Inhibition of phenolsulphotransferase P by certain food constituents. *The Lancet* **1** (8484) 794.

Jacobsen DW (1991) Adverse reactions to benzoates and parabens. In: DD Metcalfe, HA Sampson and RA Simon (Eds) *Food Allergy: Adverse reactions to foods and food additives* (pp276–287). Oxford: Blackwell Scientific Publications.

Johnson S (2001) The multifaceted and widespread pathology of magnesium deficiency. *Medical Hypotheses* **56** (2) 163–170.

Joneja JMV (1998) *Dietary Management of Food Allergies and Intolerances* (2nd edition). Vancouver: JA Hall Publications.

Joneja JMV (2001) *Dietary Management of Food Allergies and Intolerances.* Personal communication: more information available from the author.

Kaplan BJ, McNicol J, Conte RA and Moghadam HK (1989) Dietary replacement in preschool-aged hyperactive boys. *Pediatrics* **83** (1) 7–17.

Kroyer G (1986) Interaction of artificial food colours with vitamin C; and effects on enzyme activity (amylase, pepsin, trypsin). *Ernaehrung/Nutrition* (Technical University, Vienna) **10** (6) 465–467.

McCann D, Barrett A, Cooper A, Crumpler D, Dalen L, Grimshaw K, Kitchin E, Lok K, Porteous L, Prince E, Sonuga-Barke E, Warner JO and Stevenson J (2007) Food additives and hyperactive behaviour in 3-year old and 8/9-year old children in the community: a randomized, double-blinded, placebo-controlled trial. *The Lancet* **370** (9598) 1560–1567.

Millstone E (1997) Adverse reactions to food additives: the extent and severity of the problem. *Journal of Nutritional and Environmental Medicine* **7** (4) 323–332.

News of the World (2002) Dye-Cing with death, 22 July. Available at: www.kingjamestruth.co.uk/E124.htm [accessed 28/04/08].

Reyes FG, Valim MF and Vercesi AE (1996) Effect of organic synthetic food colors on mitochondrial respiration. *Food Additives and Contaminants* **13** (1) 5–11.

Rowe KS and Rowe KJ (1994) Synthetic food colouring and behaviour: a dose response effect in a double-blind, placebo controlled repeated-measures study. *Journal of Pediatrics* **125** (5) 691–698.

Sasaki YF, Kawaguchi S, Kamaya A, Ohshita M, Kabasawa K, Iwama K, Taniguchi K and Tsuda S (2002) The comet assay with eight mouse organs. *Mutation Research* **519** (1–2) 103–119.

Swanson JM and Kinsbourne M (1980) Food dyes impair performance of hyperactive children on a laboratory learning test. *Science* **207** (4438) 1485–1487.

Ward NI (1997) Assessment of chemical factors in relation to child hyperactivity. *Journal of Nutritional and Environmental Medicine* **7** (4) 333–342.

Ward NI, Soulsbury KA, Zettel VH, Colquhoun ID, Bunday S and Barnes B (1990) The influence of the chemical additive tartrazine on the zinc status of hyperactive children – a double-blind placebo controlled study. *Journal of Nutritional Medicine* **1** (1) 51–57.

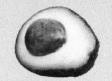

Chapter 4
The effect of mercury on the body and brain
PROFESSOR VERA STEJSKAL

Most people are exposed to low concentrations of metals on a daily basis and it is therefore surprising that researchers have not focused on how this affects health. Some metals, such as zinc and iron, are essential for human health, while many others, like mercury and lead, have no role in the human body. Since the ban of leaded petrol, mercury pollution is the biggest concern to health and the environment worldwide. The main exposure to mercury is through dental amalgam, according to World Health Organization *Environmental Health Criteria* (1991). For this reason, this article will concentrate on the mercury issue, despite the fact that other metals such as lead, manganese and arsenic can cause neurotoxicity and other health problems (Wright and Baccarelli, 2007). In addition to dental amalgam, polluted fish is a source of methylmercury and cigarette smoke contains many metals such as mercury, cadmium, nickel, lead and arsenic. Some adult vaccines and pharmaceutical preparations such as eye drops still contain the mercury preservative thimerosal.

The danger of heavy and transition metals resides in their physicochemical properties; they bind to sulphur and other groups in the mitochondria, enzymes and cell proteins. Fat-containing organs, such as brain or collagen-containing structures, are especially rich in sulphur groups and therefore vulnerable to metal binding. Metals also induce free-radical formation and inactivate enzyme and mitochondrial activity (Nuttal, 2004).

The effect of high concentrations of metals on the brain and mental health has been thoroughly studied in occupationally exposed workers. It has been established that metals such as mercury and lead are toxic to nerve cells. Acute intoxication from mercury leads to (among other symptoms) loss of appetite, weight and hair loss, severe hypertension and personality changes. Acute mercury poisoning is fortunately infrequent and mainly affects specific professions, such as miners, or people living in polluted areas, for example, through a factory's wastewater.

Health authorities in the UK stand by their claim that amalgam fillings are absolutely safe and there is no reason to replace functioning fillings. It does not seem to matter that mercury has recently been banned in Norway and Sweden. The argument is that the mercury released from fillings is below a 'safe level' established in the occupational environment. A review of current scientific literature does show that a chronic, low-dose exposure to metals can cause health problems. Before discussing the specific studies reporting the connection between metals and mental health, it is necessary to mention a common misunderstanding when it comes to exposure to metals such as mercury: *the importance to distinguish between toxic and immunological effects.* Toxic effects occur at high levels, such as in working or other accidents when a whole area is polluted, and are thankfully rather rare. Immunological effects, such as allergy or autoimmunity, can occur only in susceptible, genetically predisposed subjects and in those cases even very small amounts of the offending substance are sufficient for the development of ill health.

The role of iron and other metals in neurodegenerative diseases, such as Parkinson's, Alzheimer's and multiple sclerosis, is now firmly established (Campbell *et al*, 2001). Depression is a risk factor for neurological, as well as cardiovascular and allergic, diseases. The common factor in all these conditions is inflammation and there is a connection between inflammation in the body and some cases of depression (Dantzer *et al*, 2008). This causal relationship was first described 20 years ago and is only now starting to receive attention (McDonald *et al*, 1987). After activation, inflammatory cells release cytokines, which affect the brain through deregulation of the hypothalamic-pituitary-adrenal axis (HPA). This system is a part of the neuroendocrine system that controls vital functions, such as digestion, immune system and energy usage, but also mood and reaction to stress. Deregulation leads to multi-symptoms, including profound fatigue, fibromyalgia, psychosomatic problems and sleep disturbances (Turnbull and Rivier, 1995). Furthermore, psychological stress may not only cause immune activation, it may also result in immunosuppression (Maes, 1999).

Current medicine treats the inflammation underlying diseases, but does not generally look for the cause of inflammation. Recognised causes of inflammation are bacteria and viruses. Metals are often overlooked, however, as metal-induced inflammation (allergy) is usually regarded only as a skin disease or a local oral problem, and not as systemic disease. In addition, metals cause inflammation only in some individuals, and not in all exposed subjects.

Scientific literature is full of evidence of 'mercury poisoned' people whose symptoms disappeared after removing their fillings (Prochazkova *et al*, 2004; Stejskal *et al*, 1999; Wojcik *et al*, 2006). Since mercury is usually not regarded as an allergen, it is not surprising that most dentists are not aware of the fact that *even low concentrations of mercury as well as other dental metals (nickel, gold, palladium) might be harmful for allergic patients.*

When approached, most dentists will reject their patient's suspicion that mercury in amalgam fillings is making them sick, saying there is no proof and no laboratory tests showing that they are 'poisoned'. The problem is the term 'poisoned'. If patients said they are allergic to mercury, they might, possibly, be taken seriously. The British Dental Association admits that there are people who are allergic to metals found in amalgam fillings and that these people should have their fillings removed. They also stress that such a reaction is very rare.

Allergy to metals is mainly measured by patch/skin testing, which measures cellular type IV hypersensitivity. This involves stimulating certain types of white blood cells – T-lymphocytes – with metals. Serum factors, so-called antibodies, are absent. In contrast to a type I allergy, which is mediated by serum IgE antibodies, a type IV allergic reaction is mediated by T memory cells (white blood cells previously sensitised to given allergen). Following renewed exposure, memory lymphocytes will recognise the allergen and divide. The newly formed cells secrete cytokines and participate in the resulting allergic reaction. In patch testing, the suspected allergen is applied on the skin of the back and redness and swelling two to three days later is taken as an evidence of a positive response. Although it is the gold standard in dermatology, this test suffers from several disadvantages, such as risk of sensitisation by direct application of a toxin on the skin and low reproducibility of subjective reading.

Diagnostic tests include blood and urine testing and hair analysis and are based on the excretion of toxic metals from the body. If a person is not excreting the metal due to a lack of detoxification enzymes for example, these tests can be misleading (Nuttal, 2004).

A blood test that can measure allergy to metals outside the body (in vitro) has been available since the 1960s. The lymphocyte transformation test (LTT) was initially not standardised and therefore had low clinical relevance. In the 1990s, however, two modifications of this test were developed, the beryllium LTT test and the LTT-MELISA® test, which are now accepted methods of evaluating an allergy to metals (Newman, 1996; Stejskal *et al*, 2006; Valentine-Thon and Schiwara, 2003, Valentine-Thon *et al*, 2006). According to patch test results, inorganic mercury and thimerosal are the most frequent allergens in children, together with nickel. In 1,094 Italian children with eczema and dermatitis, 10% reacted to thimerosal and six per cent to mercury (Seidenari *et al*, 2005). In Spain, skin test reactivity to thimerosal was 21% and to mercury 19% (Vozmediano and Hita, 2005). A high prevalence of allergy to mercury was also found in LTT-MELISA® in patients with chronic fatigue syndrome (CFS) like symptoms (Stejskal *et al*, 1999) and in patients with autoimmune disorders (Prochazkova *et al*, 2004) who improved following replacement of dental amalgam.

Neuropsychiatric performances in workers occupationally exposed to mercury

The air at Ground Zero following 11 September 2001 was heavily polluted with metals and chemicals from the destroyed World Trade Centre, and service personnel and residents of Lower Manhattan inhaled these particles for an extended period of time. A study on 160 subjects found that most individuals had eight or more serious health complaints, including:

- severe respiratory problems
- digestive problems

- skin rashes
- sleeplessness
- anxiety
- depression
- weight gain
- elevated blood pressure
- lethargy
- recurrent headaches.

Heavy metal toxicity was suspected as a causal factor for many of these symptoms. Of those tested for heavy metal toxicity using a challenge urine test, 85% had excessively high levels of lead and mercury. Patients were treated by chelation using dimercaptosuccinic acid (DMSA). Chelators, from the Greek word *chelos*, meaning claw, are substances that bind tightly to metals and remove them from the body. After three to four months of treatment, the first cohort of 100 individuals reported significant (greater than 60%) improvement in all symptoms (Kokayi *et al*, 2006).

Another study looked at the neuropsychological performances of 26 ex-workers at a fluorescent lamp factory with chronic mercury poisoning. The workers had been exposed to mercury for an average of 10 years and had been away from this work for approximately six years. Twenty control subjects matched for age, gender and education were used for comparison. The neuropsychological performances of the former workers suggest that occupational exposure to elemental mercury has long-term effects on information processing and psychomotor function, with increased depression and anxiety (Zachi *et al*, 2007).

Further studies have shown that miners exposed to mercury vapour during a period of three years had intellectual damage, emotional changes (symptoms of depression and anxiety) and neurological changes (amnesia, insomnia and tremor of the tongue), as compared to miners who were not exposed to this vapour (Tirado *et al*, 2000). Ex-miners also tend to be more introverted, depressive and rigid in expressing their emotions and are likely to have more negative self-concepts than controls (Kobal *et al*, 2006).

Neuropsychiatric studies on the effects of chronic low-dose exposure to mercury released from dental amalgam

Studies of the effects of chronic low-dose exposure to mercury released from amalgam fillings are less frequent than the epidemiologic studies of workers, but show similar health outcomes. The occurrence of neuropsychiatric symptoms, such as fatigue, insomnia, anxiety and anger in 25 women who had amalgam fillings was compared with 23 women without amalgams. The women with amalgams had significantly higher levels of mercury in the saliva and showed more symptoms of fatigue and insomnia. They experienced more intense, angry feelings and were significantly less pleasant, satisfied, happy, secure and steady, and found it more difficult to make decisions. The study suggests that mercury released from amalgam may be an etiological factor in depression, excessive anger, and anxiety, perhaps because mercury affects neurotransmitters in the brain (Siblerud *et al*, 1994).

The same group of scientists studied the smoking habits of 119 subjects without amalgam fillings and compared them with 115 subjects with amalgams. The amalgam group had 2.5 times more smokers per group than the non-amalgam group, which was highly significant. Mercury decreases dopamine, serotonin, norepinephrine and acetylcholine in the brain and nicotine has just the opposite effect on these neurotransmitters, which may help to explain why people with dental amalgams smoke more than people without amalgams (Siblerud *et al*, 1993).

Finally, the mental health status of 47 multiple sclerosis patients with amalgams was compared with that of 50 patients who had their fillings removed. Multiple sclerosis subjects with amalgams suffered significantly more depression, hostility and psychotic behaviour and were more obsessive-compulsive than the patients with removed fillings. These data suggested that the poorer mental health status exhibited by multiple sclerosis subjects with amalgam fillings may be associated with mercury toxicity from the amalgam (Siblerud, 1992).

The beneficial effect of replacement of dental amalgam in patients suffering from various allergic and autoimmune diseases has been confirmed in more recent studies (Prochazkova *et al*, 2004; Sterzl *et al*, 2006; Stejskal *et al*, 2006; Valentine-Thon *et al*, 2006).

Biochemical markers of mercury-susceptible populations

In a New Zealand study already mentioned above (Wojcik *et al*, 2006), 465 patients were diagnosed as having chronic mercury toxicity according to well-established criteria. Thirty-two per cent of patients suffered from severe fatigue, 89% had memory loss and 28% had depression. A significant correlation was found between a special variant of apo-lipoprotein E gene and increased amalgam susceptibility, indicating that genetic factors may play a role. Removal of amalgam mercury fillings combined with chelation and antioxidant treatment resulted in significant symptom reduction ($p<0.001$) to levels reported by healthy subjects. These data confirm previously published findings from the same group (Godfrey *et al*, 2003) and of others regarding susceptibility to Alzheimer's disease (Roses, 1998) and to toxic effects of lead (Stewart *et al*, 2002). Another study looked at 309 gold miners and unexposed controls with regards to mercury concentration in body fluids. The results indicated that a special variation of the gene involved in the synthesis of glutathione (a cellular antioxidant) was present in individuals who had increased blood, plasma and urine levels of mercury. Since glutathione is used for detoxification of mercury and other metals, subjects with decreased glutathione availability might have problems with the detoxicification of mercury (Custodio *et al*, 2005).

Recently, a clinical study concluded that dental amalgam has no neurobehavioral effects in children (Bellinger *et al*, 2006). However, at the beginning of the study, children previously diagnosed with psychological, behavioural, neurological or immunological disorders were eliminated from the studied group. One wonders if these children might have been susceptible to amalgam. Any lack of effects in healthy children should not exclude possible effects in susceptible ones. Future studies should, therefore, not just be performed on a random population, but in groups with suspected sensitivity to mercury, such as people with mercury allergy or a problem with detoxification. Their health should be monitored before and after safe amalgam replacement.

The involvement of toxic metals in the origin of disease has been known for 20 years (Grandjean, 2008) and, so far, the application of new scientific knowledge in clinical practice has been painfully slow. The availability of new laboratory tests enables susceptible groups to be identified and treated earlier.

Conclusion

Mercury has strong toxic and allergenic properties. In addition to acute toxicity experienced in occupationally exposed workers, susceptible groups, such as those with an allergic predisposition and autoimmune disorders, might be especially prone to low doses of mercury.

In people chronically exposed to low doses of mercury, testing for levels of mercury in blood, urine or hair usually does not show whether the metal is causing disease. Allergy to mercury and other metals can be determined at dermatology clinics by patch test or blood testing with LTT-MELISA®. Genetic testing has not yet been used outside the occupational setting, but may be a promising option in the future.

In allergic individuals, exposure to mercury and other toxic substances should be eliminated. Any removal of amalgam fillings has to be done by an informed dentist following maximal protection against mercury exposure. Non-metallic dental materials should be used, such as composites and ceramics. Detoxification and antioxidant treatment with minerals and vitamins counteracting the effect of mercury and other metals may be prescribed by a physician or a qualified nutritional therapist.

References

Bellinger DC, Trachtenberg F, Barregard L, Tavares M, Cernichiari E, Daniel D and McKinlay S (2006) Neuropsychological and renal effects of dental amalgam in children: a randomized clinical trial. *JAMA* **295** (15) 1775–1783.

Campbell A, Smith MA, Sayre LM, Bondy SC and Perry G (2001) Mechanisms by which metals promote events connected to neurodegenerative diseases. *Brain Research Bulletin* **55** (2) 125–132.

Custodio HM, Harari R, Gerhardsson L, Skerfving S and Broberg K (2005) Genetic influences on the retention of inorganic mercury. *Archives of Environmental and Occupational Health* **60** (1) 17–23.

Dantzer R, O'Connor JC, Freund GG, Johnson RW and Kelley KW (2008) From inflammation to sickness and depression: when the immune system subjugates the brain. *Nature Reviews: Neuroscience* **9** (1) 46–56.

Godfrey M, Wojcik DP and Krone CA (2003) Apolipoprotein E genotyping as a potential biomarker for mercury neurotoxicity. *Journal of Alzheimer's Disease* **5** (3) 189–195.

Grandjean P (2008) Late insights into early origins of disease. *Basic and Clinical Pharmacology and Toxicology* **102** (2) 94–99.

Kobal GD, Kobal AB, Arneric N, Horvat M and Zenko B (2006) Personality traits in miners with past occupational elemental mercury exposure. *Environmental Health Perspectives* **114** (2) 290–296.

Kokayi K, CH Altman , RW Callely and A Harrison (2006) Findings of and treatment for high levels of mercury and lead toxicity in ground zero rescue and recovery workers and lower Manhattan residents. *Explore (New York)* **2** (5) 400–407.

Maes M (1999) Psychological stress, cytokines, and the inflammatory response system. *Current Opinion in Psychiatry* **12** (6) 697–700.

McDonald EM, Mann AH and Thomas HC (1987) Interferons as mediators of psychiatric morbidity. An investigation in a trial of recombinant alpha-interferon in hepatitis-B carriers. *The Lancet* **21** (2) 1175–1178.

Newman LS (1996) Significance of the blood beryllium lymphocyte proliferation test. *Environmental Health Perspectives* **104** (S5) 953–956.

Nuttal KL (2004) Interpreting mercury in blood and urine of individual patients. *Annals of Clinical and Laboratory Science* **34** 235–250.

Prochazkova J, Sterzl I, Kucerova H, Bartova J and Stejskal V (2004) The beneficial effect of amalgam replacement on health in patients with autoimmunity. *Neuroendocrinology Letters* **25** (3) 211–218.

Roses AD (1998) Apolipoprotein E and Alzheimer's disease: the tip of the susceptibility iceberg. *Annals of the New York Academy of Sciences* **855** (1) 738–743.

Seidenari S, Giusti F, Pepe P and Mantovani L (2005) Contact sensitization in 1094 children undergoing patch testing over a seven-year period. *Pediatric Dermatology* **22** (1) 1–5.

Siblerud RL (1992) A comparison of mental health of multiple sclerosis patients with silver/mercury dental fillings and those with fillings removed. *Psychological Reports* **70** (3) 1139–1151.

Siblerud RL, Kienholz E and Motl J (1993) Evidence that mercury from silver dental fillings may be an etiological factor in smoking. *Toxicology Letters* **68** 307–310.

Siblerud RL, Motl J and Kienholz E (1994) Psychometric evidence that mercury from silver dental fillings may be an etiological factor in depression, excessive anger, and anxiety. *Psychological Reports* **74** (1) 67–80.

Stejskal V, Danersund A, Lindvall A, Hudecek R, Nordman V, Yaqob A, Lindh U, Mayer W and Bieger W (1999) Metal-specific lymphocytes: biomarkers of sensitivity in man. *Neuroendocrinology Letters* **20** (5) 289–298.

Stejskal V, Hudecek R, Stejskal J and Sterzl I (2006) Diagnosis and treatment of metal-induced side-effects. *Neuroendocrinology Letters* **27** (S1) 7–16.

Sterzl I, Procházková J, Hrda P, Matucha P, Bartova J and Stejskal V (2006) Removal of dental amalgam decreases anti-TPO and anti-Tg autoantibodies in patients with autoimmune thyroiditis. *Neuroendocrinology Letters* **27** (S1) 25–30.

Stewart WF, Schwartz BS, Simon D, Kelsey K and Todd AC (2002) ApoE genotype past adult lead exposure and neurobehavioral function. *Environmental Health Perspective* **110** (5) 501–505.

Tirado V, Garcia MA, Moreno J, Galeano LM, Lopera F and Franco A (2000) Neuropsychological disorders after occupational exposure to mercury vapors in El Bagre (Antioquia, Colombia). *Revista de Neurología* **31** (8) 712–716.

Turnbull A and Rivier C (1995) Regulation of the HPA axis by cytokines. *Brain, Behavior, and Immunity* **9** (4) 253–275.

Valentine-Thon E, Muller K, Guzzi G, Kreisel S, Ohnsorge P and Sandkamp M (2006) LTT-MELISA is clinically relevant for detecting and monitoring metal sensitivity. *Neuroendocrinology Letters* **27** (S1) 17–24.

Valentine-Thon E and Schiwara HW (2003) Validity of MELISA® for metal sensitivity. *Neuroendocrinology Letters* 2003 **24** (1–2) 57–64.

Vozmediano JMF and Hita A (2005) Allergic contact dermatitis in children. *Journal of the European Academy of Dermatology and Venereology* **19** (S1) 42–46.

Wojcik DP, Godfrey ME, Christie D and Haley BE (2006) Mercury toxicity presenting as chronic fatigue, memory impairment and depression: diagnosis, treatment, susceptibility, and outcomes in a New Zealand general practice setting (1994–2006). *Neuroendocrinology Letters* **27** (4) 415–423.

World Health Organization (1991) *Environmental Health Criteria 118: Inorganic mercury.* Geneva: World Health Organization.

Wright RO and Baccarelli A (2007) Metals and neurotoxicity. *Journal of Nutrition* **137** (12) 2809–2813.

Zachi EC, Faria MA and Taub A (2007) Neuropsychological dysfunction related to earlier occupational exposure to mercury vapor. *Brazilian Journal of Medical and Biological Research* **40** (3) 425–433.

Chapter 5

Resolving depression: the role of the gut in taming inflammation

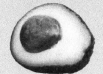

MICHAEL ASH

Depression is a global health problem; it is widespread, tends to follow a relapsing or concurrent course of action, damages and disrupts social and vocational activities and is closely linked to increased morbidity and a reduced life expectancy (Kessler *et al*, 2007). Depression has become the third most common reason for consultation in primary health care (Shah, 1992).

Over the last few centuries, approaches to treating the mentally unwell have changed dramatically. Only a few decades ago, cutting-edge therapies included lobotomies and insulin-induced states of coma; prior to these, the plunging of 'the ill' into ice-filled baths as advocated by Dr Emil Kraepelin was prescribed.

Manipulation of our neurochemistry is now the mainstay of contemporary medical practice and, while from a pharmacological perspective there have been ongoing improvements in patient outcomes, particularly through the use of the newer serotonin, dopamine and norepinephrine reuptake inhibitors (Szabo *et al*, 2004), there are still considerable limitations in their effectiveness. Less than half of all people prescribed these medications for one year will have any significant resolution of their symptoms, even when they remain compliant and live in favourable conditions (Rush *et al*, 2006). Alternatives to the pharmaceutical or behavioural approaches may, therefore, appeal to the clinician, therapist and patient.

An area of considerable attention for such a strategy involves the body's inflammatory process. Inflammation can be regarded as a silent and stressful challenge to our bodies that can effect profound behavioural change: a *'malignant flame'* that needs to be managed and extinguished to avoid collateral damage (Connor and Leonard, 2000).

Our innate immune defence

One particular immune element attracting most interest in its relationship with depression and other conditions is the 'innate' immune system. This section of our immune system actually originated over 500 million years ago, when a remarkable evolution in our natural defences developed.

Specialised proteins and enzymes, designed to defend our primitive ancestors against external assaults were created and formed. They utilise a brutal combination of strategies: punching holes in cell membranes, spitting out chemical toxins or just consuming and digesting the enemy. Following eradication of the transgressor, this system also co-ordinates repair and renewal or encourages cellular suicide when the involved cell tissues are too damaged to salvage.

So effective is this innate immune defence, that it is still in place and operational in our bodies today, acting as promoter and controller of inflammation. While until recently it was regarded by scientists as the somewhat basic and thuggish element of our immune defences, the last few years has seen a dramatic change in focus away from the memory-encoded 'adaptive' system to this ancient conserved 'innate' system (Medzhitov and Janeway, 2000). This change in attention has been driven by the incredible advances in understanding the effects of inflammation on many different diseases from diabetes, allergies, cancer, heart disease and mood disorders, including depression.

The immune system and brain share an extraordinarily intricate communication network in which immunological information travels continuously and rapidly to and from the brain and immune system to provide a range of checks and balances. A fundamental point to remember is that in a healthy person the immune system should be doing nothing except observing. We have become so focused on the immune system responding to things that we forget that, for 99.99% of the time, its job is *not* to respond (McGeer and McGeer, 2002).

The immune system operates as a diffuse sensory collecting system, transferring information to the brain about the health of our body. The brain in turn releases chemical signals to constrain and direct our immune system (Hadley, 2004). In optimal health, it is kept in a state of unresponsiveness until called on to react quickly and effectively. In ill health, however, the immune system remains switched on, consuming energy by constantly releasing inflammation promoting agents.

The role of proinflammatory cytokines

When any tissue in the body becomes chronically inflamed in response to pathogens, toxins, substance abuse, genetic damage, trauma, stress, parasitic, bacterial or fungal overgrowth, our immune system will boost the production of inflammatory proteins called cytokines. These proinflammatory cytokines increase the risk, development or maintenance of illness (Irani, 2002). People suffering from clinical depression have shown 40–50% higher concentrations of proinflammatory cytokines.

> Cytokines (eg. IL1, TNFα, IL6) are small proteins released from white blood cells that act as chemical signals between immune cells, other cells and organs, including the brain. In the immune system's attempt to maintain homeostasis, each one can either stimulate or inhibit a response depending on the presence of other cytokines and overall metabolic activity.

These inflammatory chemicals, specifically released to enhance our recovery, may enter or influence the brain and induce a change in behaviour, originally described as 'sickness behaviour'. Cytokines are associated with many of the key symptoms of depression: mood state changes, neurodevelopmental problems and even some psychiatric conditions as well as social withdrawal, loss of interest in sex, change in appetite, change in sleep patterns and anxiety (Vollmer-Conna *et al*, 2004).

The recognition that our immune system may be involved – both as a result of interaction with our social and psychological environment via 'stress' and with infection, trauma and disease, is not new. Back in 200 AD, Galen, a Greek Physician recorded that 'melancholic' women were more prone to cancer of the breast, and numerous reports in early observational and medical literature from many authors note that depression is often concomitant with bacterial or viral infections.

In the late 19th and early 20th centuries this idea was further explored by the Viennese Psychiatrist Julius Wagner-Jauregg who induced fever via bacterial substrates to influence the course of depression and schizophrenia. His work was revolutionary and controversial, earning him the Nobel Prize for medicine in 1927 (Nobel Lectures, 1965).

The second half of the 20th century and the early years of the 21st century have seen increasingly significant inroads into understanding, with more accuracy, how psychological health is both affected by, and affects, the immune system (Prolo *et al*, 2002). The evolving hypothesis that adverse psychological states can be reversed by the resolution of immune disturbances is gaining credibility as an area of great therapeutic potential and is viewed as a new frontier in treatment prospects (Roy-Byrne, 2006).

In 1995 the first paper exploring the concept of 'cytokine-induced sickness behaviour' was published (Aubert *et al*, 1995) and the years following have seen a much clearer role of cytokines beyond the acute phase of infection or stress in creating altered psychological health (Dantzer and Kelley, 2007).

CYTOKINES: MASTER REGULATORS OF THE IMMUNE SYSTEM

- You cannot experience an emotion or think a thought without biological correlates.
- You cannot experience a biological correlate without an immune activation.
- You cannot experience an immune activation without the release and binding of cytokines.

It is, of course, easier and almost instinctive for us to accept that our psychological health is linked to psychosocial or 'stressful experiences' rather than determined, to a degree, by our immune system. Yet, a subset of people with depression develop and sustain depression due to immune activation and the subsequent and ongoing production of proinflammatory cytokines (Theoharides *et al*, 2004). It should be noted that stress, in itself, is a powerful immune inflammation activating event (Chrousos, 2000).

The association between depression and inflammation is apparent even in mild depressive symptoms, including individual symptoms, such as fatigue, anger, sleep disturbances and anhedonia (an inability to experience pleasure from normally pleasurable life events such as eating, exercise and social or sexual interaction) (Suarez *et al*, 2004; Suarez *et al*, 2002; Maier and Watkins, 1998). However, not everyone who has an altered immune response will display depressive behaviour. People have distinct variations in their responses to these inflammatory messengers.

So how might these cytokines access the brain? Three well-defined mechanisms offer rational explanations.

1. They cross leaky regions of the blood–brain barrier.
2. They are carried by specialist molecules across the blood–brain barrier.
3. They are transported via the vagal nerve.

Cytokines can, but do not have to, enter the brain directly to have an effect as they can stimulate the release of secondary chemicals that amplify the effect of existing cytokines in the brain (Dantzer, 2004).

Cytokines interfere with the dominant neurotransmitters, serotonin, dopamine and norepinephrine – the key targets of today's pharmaceutical approach (Dunn, 1999). Although they stimulate key hormones used by the body to mitigate stress, they can also increase anxiety and fear (Silverman *et al*, 2005).

One other pivotal inflammatory controlling agent called nuclear factor kappa B (NFkB) is activated by cytokines. This agent contributes to the slow repair of neuronal tissues, reducing the normal plasticity of brain repair and inducing oxidative stress, all of which are linked to depressive behaviour (Madrigal *et al*, 2002).

The gut–brain link

Functional gastrointestinal problems, such as irritable bowel syndrome, are commonly linked to anxiety and mood changes (Dunlop *et al*, 2003). The GI tract has over 100 million neurons and has the second largest collection of neural tissue in the body (after the brain) called the enteric nervous system (ENS).

The mucosal tissues, such as those in the gut, represent the largest part of our body's innate immune system and the most likely tissue for altered immune activity. The first point of contact for possible pathogens is the GI tract, lungs or some other part of the body – not the brain. Defence cells produce their cytokines at the site of infection.

The mind and body work as an integrated unit to promote survival and recovery during infection or trauma. Indeed, developmental studies have now demonstrated that when the innate immune system is activated, it can induce depression independent of sickness, meaning that stress itself is an activator and then responder to innate immune chemicals (Frenois *et al*, 2006). Not everyone, of course, responds to inflammation as a depressive trigger, or even to the same severity. This difference in sensitivity depends on genes, hormones, diet, medication, gender and the environmental and emotional exposures experienced in utero and in early life.

Growing evidence shows that our sensitivity to stress as adults is already 'dialled in' in infancy. Essentially, the level of stress encountered in early life sensitises us to a certain level of adversity. High levels of early life stress can result in hypersensitivity to stress as well as adult depression later, due to changes to our stress response network (Licinio and Wong, 1999).

'A history of various stressors such as abuse and neglect in early life as well as foetal stress and nutrient depletion are a common feature of early life in those with chronic depression in adulthood.' (Jablensky, 2005)

Of great interest to clinicians has been that this group of inflammation-sensitive depressives tends not to respond to anti-depressive medication. They fall into the atypical pattern of depression with a blunted stress response and a tendency to gain weight. Other conditions where this pattern may be seen include chronic fatigue, seasonal affective disorder and fibromyalgia (Wallace, 2001).

The gastrointestinal tract is a site of great clinical interest as events that affect the immune system are transferred via cytokine activation along the vagal nerve to the brain in milliseconds. All receptors found in the brain are also found in the gut, making the information exchange fast and direct. Infection, stress and trauma, as well as ongoing gastrointestinal problems, will provide a constant source of neural inflammation. The question is, therefore, can the gastrointestinal tract be used to send anti-inflammatory signals to the brain to compete with, and neutralise, provocative proinflammatory cytokines?

The use of nutritional and microbial agents to reduce inflammation and promote our natural anti-inflammatory responses is attracting considerable attention, for their low risk-to-benefit ratio and ease of use. The next section will explore some of the more refined strategies used by clinicians employing nutritional medicine.

NFkB inhibition

NFkB is a chemical that amplifies the effect of inflammation by activating over 400 genes specially encoded for inflammation. It represents an area of significant investigation for the control of inflammation. There is little evidence of health gain in switching it off altogether, but a number of natural agents found in our foods and supplements have been safely used for hundreds of years to provide a reasonable level of control over this important mechanism.

The use of vitamins C, E and N-acetylcysteine (Pajonk, 2002), cat's claw extract (Akesson, 2003), green and black tea polyphenols (Pan *et al*, 2000), the spice curcumin (Kumar, 1998), citrus flavonoids (Chen *et al*, 2004) and others have all shown NFkB-inhibiting effects (Bremner and Heinrich, 2002).

Maintaining control over NFkB, together with other anti-inflammatory strategies (such as suitable food selection and probiotic therapy), represents a sensible evidence-based route for resolving inflammation-related depression.

Probiotics as inflammation controllers

Anti-inflammatory cytokines are used and produced by the commensal bacteria to maintain immune tolerance in the gastrointestinal tract. They do this by using codes in their membranes that are recognised by the innate immune system as being friend rather than foe. Knowing that certain types of bacteria induce anti-inflammatory responses, allows us to introduce bacteria into the gastrointestinal tract to affect inflammation both locally and systemically (by a process known as bystander suppression) and thereby affect mood. Certain bacteria also reduce activation of NFkB, providing a double-edged benefit (Neu *et al*, 2007).

Research suggests that bacteria in the gastrointestinal tract can communicate with the central nervous system, even in the absence of an immune response (Eutamene and Bueno, 2007). We also know that stress, a significant factor in depression, alters the balance of intestinal bacteria by lowering the levels of lactobacilli and *Bifidobacterium* (Lyte and Bailey, 1997; Kinney *et al*, 2000).

Probiotics are able to lower systemic inflammatory cytokines, decrease oxidative stress and improve nutritional status. When used correctly, they have the potential to be significant players in the management of inflammation-induced depression.

Probiotics also play an important role in the production of a special immune cell called a regulatory T cell. These cells act as the 'peace keepers' of the immune system. They are made in small numbers in the thymus, but in great numbers in the gastrointestinal tract. The cells can travel from the gastrointestinal tract around the body, calming down inflammation and also act to encourage the production of anti-inflammatory cytokines through their controlling influence over our gastrointestinal bacterial composition and their support of the adaptive immune system (Sakaguchi, 2004).

Our bodies produce only one type of anti-inflammatory immunoglobulin and this is called secretory IgA (sIgA). We manufacture more of this than any other immune chemical and it is produced mainly in the gastrointestinal tract. As well as modifying inflammation, it is essential in helping bacteria to survive and to deliver their encoded message. However, sIgA is very susceptible to emotion and frustration, which will lower its production dramatically (Bosch *et al*, 2007). The use of probiotics and introduction of a friendly yeast called *Saccharomyces boulardii* will enhance sIgA production, so reducing immune-promoted inflammation in the mucosal tissues (Fooks and Gibson, 2002).

Saccharomyces boulardii is a tropical strain of yeast first isolated from lychee and mangosteen fruit by French scientist Henri Boulard (Malgoire *et al*, 2005). It is a transient resident of the gastrointestinal tract but has the ability to reduce inflammation and increase our natural anti-inflammatory sIgA production (Dahan *et al*, 2003; Buts *et al*, 1990).

Probiotics are live (not freeze dried) microbes that, when delivered in adequate amounts, confer a health benefit to the consumer (Food and Agriculture Organization/World Health Organization, 2001). Studies have demonstrated superior activity of live compared with killed probiotics, in in vitro and in human studies (Zhang, 2005; Cruchet *et al*, 2003; Gotteland *et al*, 2001). Even though not all studies show an advantage to viability (Peng and Hsu, 2005; Rachmilewitz *et al*, 2004), probiotics, by definition, must be administered alive. There is another particularly important consideration for probiotics: different strains of species of bacteria have different functions. The selection of strain for inflammation management, rather than incremental increase, is of vital clinical importance. Large strain-specific differences in immunopotential have been observed among different strains of the same *Bifidobacterium* species.

The required dose is dependent on a variety of factors, including physiological characteristics of strains being used, types of clinical endpoints being tracked, whether the endpoint is prophylactic or therapeutic, length of time of administration of probiotic, the prior health of the GI tract, and other bioactive ingredients used in conjunction with the probiotic.

Indoleamine and mood

When our immune system is activated against infection, trauma or under stress, we release indoleamine 2,3-dioxygenase (IDO). This is a tryptophan-metabolising enzyme, which has been part of immune defence for the past 600 million years. IDO has a key role in controlling adaptive immune responses, chronic infections, allergy and auto immunity and has a role to play in depression (Grohmann *et al*, 2003; Mellor and Munn, 2004; Sharma *et al*, 2007).

During inflammation IDO inhibits tryptophan conversion to the mood-aiding neurotransmitter serotonin. While the aim of this process is to starve certain bacteria of tryptophan as food, the consequence is prolonged inflammation and a loss of available serotonin, further contributing to depressive behaviour. At the same time, the re-uptake of serotonin is blocked by other inflammatory chemicals, so that the longer the inflammation remains, the less serotonin is available.

In addition, IDO-potent neurotoxin by-products (quinolinic, picolinic acid, kynurenines) are implicated in altered neurological function as well as depression (Leonard, 2007; Müller and Schwarz, 2007). Finally, IDO limits the biosynthesis of nicotinic acid (B3), a vitamin essential for adrenal hormones and serotonin production, further contributing to risk of stress, inflammation and depression.

Mood boosters

Folate and B12 deficiency (Coppen and Bolander-Gouaille, 2005), common through poor food selection, also contribute to the symptoms of depression (Alpert and Fava, 1997) and poor response to antidepressants (Bowers and Reynolds, 1972). A vitamin B complex supplement containing all the B vitamins, therefore, has clinical justification.

The use of essential fatty acids has been found to have a variety of effects on mood and depression, including the specific reduction of depression linked to proinflammatory cytokines (Song *et al*, 2003). The consumption of cold-pressed olive oil has also been linked to a reduction of key inflammatory molecules (Beauchamp *et al*, 2005).

A summary of practical nutritional approaches

Poor food selection will contribute to the increased level of circulating inflammatory cytokines, beyond the association with increased gastrointestinal tract permeability.

Avoid

- Rancid polyunsaturated and partly hydrogenated fats and oils. These fats lead to the production of pro-inflammatory prostaglandins and should be eliminated from the diet. However, these fats are found in most processed foods or fast foods and are hard to avoid, meaning that food selection and meal planning need to be organised and should exclude an excess of pre-prepared foods.

- Olive oil can be used as an alternative to margarine or shortening. Olive oil contains omega-9 fatty acids, which work with omega-3 essential fatty acids to increase its benefits on the body, including the reduction of depressive symptoms.

Include

- Good fats in the diet are omega-3 fatty acids, found mainly in fish of cold-water origin, such as mackerel, salmon, sardines, anchovies and herring. Omega-3 fatty acids can also be found in walnuts, Brazil nuts, almonds, pumpkin seeds and sunflower seeds.

- Foods that have anti-inflammatory properties include fruits, vegetables, wholegrains, nuts and seeds. Fruits and vegetables include blackberries, strawberries, raspberries, kiwi, peaches, mango, melon, apples, carrots, squash, sweet potato, spinach, kale, greens, broccoli, cabbage and brussel sprouts. Grains include lentils, chickpeas, brown rice, wheat germ and non-instant oatmeal. These food items are also high in vitamins A, C and E.

■ Two other important components to the anti-inflammatory diet are ginger and turmeric.

A suggested list of nutritional supplements/strategies

1. Consume probiotics of bifido bacteria and lactic acid bacteria. Continue taking these for many months as it takes considerable time for the immune system in the gastrointestinal tract to be reprogrammed.
2. *Saccharomyces boulardii.*
3. Quality fish oils (EPA/DHA).
4. Natural inhibitors of NFkB.
5. Eat an anti-inflammatory diet.
6. Test for and remove any intestinal pathogens.

It is highly recommended that advice from a suitably qualified and experienced nutritional therapist is sought prior to trying out any of the above recommendations.

References

Akesson C (2003) An extract of *Uncaria tomentosa* inhibiting cell division and NF-kappa B activity without inducing cell death. *International Immunopharmacology* **3** (13–14) 1889–1900.

Alpert JE and Fava M (1997) Nutrition and depression: the role of folate. *Nutrition Review* **55** (5) 145–149.

Aubert A, Vega C, Dantzer R and Goodall G (1995) Pyrogens specifically disrupt the acquisition of a task involving cognitive processing in the rat. *Brain, Behavior, and Immunity* **9** (2) 129–148.

Beauchamp GK, Keast RS, Morel D, Lin J, Pika J, Han Q, Lee CH, Smith AB and Breslin PA (2005) Phytochemistry: ibuprofen-like activity in extra-virgin olive oil. *Nature* **437** (7055) 45–46.

Bosch JA, Engeland CG, Cacioppo JT and Marucha PT (2007) Depressive symptoms predict mucosal wound healing. *Psychosomatic Medicine* **69** (7) 597–605.

Bowers MB Jr and Reynolds EH (1972) Cerebrospinal-fluid folate and acid monoamine metabolites. *The Lancet* **2** (7791) 1376.

Bremner P and Heinrich M (2002) Natural products as targeted modulators of the nuclear factor-kappaB pathway. *Journal of Pharmacy and Pharmacology* **54** (4) 453–472.

Buts JP, Bernasconi P, Vaerman JP and Dive C (1990) Stimulation of secretory IgA and secretory component of immunoglobulins in small intestine of rats treated with *Saccharomyces boulardii. Digestive Diseases Sciences* **35** (2) 251–256.

Chen CC, Chow MP, Huang WC, Lin YC and Chang YJ (2004) Flavonoids inhibit tumor necrosis factor-alpha-induced up-regulation of intercellular adhesion molecule-1 (ICAM-1) in respiratory epithelial cells through activator protein-1 and nuclear factor-kappaB: structure-activity relationships. *Molecular Pharmacology* **66** (3) 683–693.

Chrousos GP (2000) The stress response and immune function: clinical implications. The 1999 Novera H Spector Lecture. *Annals of the New York Academy of Sciences* **917** 38–67.

Connor TJ and Leonard BE (2000) Depression, stress and immunological activation: the role of cytokines in depressive disorders. *Life Sciences* **62** (7) 583–606.

Coppen A and Bolander-Gouaille CJ (2005) Treatment of depression: time to consider folic acid and vitamin B12. *Journal of Psychopharmacology* **19** (1) 59–65.

Cruchet S, Obregon MC, Salazar G, Diaz E and Gotteland M (2003) Effect of the ingestion of a dietary product containing *Lactobacillus johnsonii* La1 on *Helicobacter pylori* colonisation in children. *Nutrition* **19** (9) 716–721.

Dahan S, Dalmasso G, Imbert V, Peyron JF, Rampal P and Czerucka D (2003) *Saccharomyces boulardii* interferes with enterohemorrhagic *Escherichia coli*-induced signaling pathways in T84 cells. *Infection and Immunity* **71** (2) 766–773.

Dantzer R (2004) Cytokine-induced sickness behaviour: a neuroimmune response to activation of innate immunity. *European Journal of Pharmacology* **500** (1–3) 399–411.

Dantzer R and Kelley KW (2007) Twenty years of research on cytokine-induced sickness behavior. *Brain, Behavior, and Immunity* **21** (2) 153–160.

Dunlop SP, Jenkins D, Neal KR and Spiller RC (2003) Relative importance of enterochromaffin cell hyperplasia, anxiety, and depression in post infectious IBS. *Gastroenterology* **125** (6) 1651–1659.

Dunn AJ (1999) Effects of cytokines on cerebral neurotransmission. Comparison with the effects of stress. *Advances in Experimental Medicine and Biology* **461** 117–127.

Eutamene H and Bueno L (2007) Role of probiotics in correcting abnormalities of colonic flora induced by stress. *Gut* **56** (11) 1495–1497.

Food and Agriculture Organization/World Health Organization (2001) *Health and Nutritional Properties of Probiotics in Food including Powder Milk with Live Lactic Acid Bacteria*. Available at: www.who.int/foodsafety/publications/fs_management/en/probiotics.pdf [accessed 28/04/08].

Fooks LJ and GR Gibson (2002) Probiotics as modulators of the gastrointestinal tract flora. *British Journal of Nutrition* **88** (S1) 39–49.

Frenois F, Moreau M, Micon C, Lestage J, Kelley KW, Dantzer R and Castanon N (2006) Lipopolysaccharide induces delayed cellular activities within the mouse extended amygdala, hippocampus and hypothalamus that parallel the expression of depressive-like behaviour in mice. *Psychoneuroendocrinology* **32** (5) 516–531.

Gotteland M, Cruchet S and Verbeke S (2001) Effect of *Lactobacillus* ingestion on the gastrointestinal mucosal barrier alterations induced by indometacin in humans. *Alimentary Pharmacology and Therapeutics* **15** (1) 11–17.

Grohmann U, Fallarino F and Puccetti P (2003) Tolerance, DCs and tryptophan: much ado about IDO. *Trends in Immunology* **24** (5) 242–248.

Hadley C (2004) Should auld acquaintance be forgot... *EMBO Reports* **5** (12) 1122–1124.

Irani DN (2002) How much control does the brain exert over the immune system? *Current Opinion in Neurology* **15** (3) 323–326.

Jablensky AV (2005) Pregnancy, delivery, and neonatal complications in a population cohort of women with schizophrenia and major affective disorders. *American Journal of Psychiatry* **162** (1) 79–91.

Kessler RC, Merikangas KR and Wang PS (2007) Prevalence, comorbidity, and service utilization for mood disorders in the United States at the beginning of the twenty-first century. *Annual Review of Clinical Psychology* **3** 137–158.

Kinney KS, Austin CE, Morton DS and Sonnenfeld G (2000) Norepinephrine as a growth stimulating factor in bacteria-mechanistic studies. *Life Sciences* **67** (25) 3075–3085.

Kumar A (1998) Curcumin (diferuloylmethane) inhibition of tumor necrosis factor (TNF)-mediated adhesion of monocytes to endothelial cells by suppression of cell surface expression of adhesion molecules and of nuclear factor-kappaB activation. *Biochemical Pharmacology* **55** (6) 775–783.

Leonard BE (2007) Inflammation, depression and dementia: are they connected? *Neurochemical Research* **32** (10) 1749–1756.

Licinio J and Wong ML (1999) The role of inflammatory mediators in the biology of major depression: central nervous system cytokines modulate the biological substrate of depressive symptoms, regulate stress-responsive systems, and contribute to neurotoxicity and neuroprotection. *Molecular Psychiatry* **4** (4) 317–327.

Lyte M and Bailey MT (1997) Neuroendocrine-bacterial interactions in a neurotoxin-induced model of trauma. *Journal of Surgical Research* **70** (2) 195–201.

Madrigal JLM, Hurtado O, Moro MA, Lizasoain I, Lorenzo P, Castrillo A, Bosca L and Leza JC (2002) The increase in TNF-alpha levels is implicated in NF-kappaB activation and inducible nitric oxide synthase expression in brain cortex after immobilization stress. *Neuropsychopharmacology* **26** (2) 155–163.

Maier SF and Watkins LR (1998) Cytokines for psychologists: implications of bidirectional immune-to-brain communication for understanding behaviour, mood, and cognition. *Psychological Review* **105** (1) 83–107.

Malgoire JY, Bertout S, Renaud F, Bastide JM and Mallié M (2005) Typing of *Saccharomyces cerevisiae* clinical strains by using microsatellite sequence polymorphism. *Journal of Clinical Microbiology* **43** (3) 1133–1137.

McGeer PL and McGeer EG (2002) Innate immunity, local inflammation, and degenerative disease. *Science of Aging Knowledge Environment* **29** (3).

Medzhitov R and Janeway C Jr (2000) Innate immunity. *The New England Journal of Medicine* **343** (5) 338–344.

Mellor AL and Munn DH (2004) IDO expression by dendritic cells: tolerance and tryptophan catabolism. *Nature Reviews Immunology* **4** (10) 762–774.

Müller N and Schwarz MJ (2007) The immune-mediated alteration of serotonin and glutamate: towards an integrated view of depression. *Molecular Psychiatry* **12** (11) 988–1000.

Neu J, Douglas-Escobar M and Lopez M (2007) Microbes and the developing gastrointestinal tract. *Nutrition in Clinical Practice* **22** (2) 174–182.

Nobel Lectures (1965) *Physiology or Medicine 1922–1941*. Amsterdam: Elsevier Publishing Company.

Pajonk F (2002) N-acetyl-L-cysteine inhibits 26S proteasome function: implications for effects on NF-kappaB activation. *Free Radical Biology and Medicine* **32** (6) 536–543.

Pan MH, Lin-Shiau SY, Ho CT, Lin JH and Lin JK (2000) Suppression of lipopolysaccharide-induced nuclear factor-kappaB activity by theaflavin-3,3'-digallate from black tea and other polyphenols through down-regulation of IkappaB kinase activity in macrophages. *Biochemical Pharmacology* **59** (4) 357–367.

Peng GC and Hsu CH (2005) The efficacy and safety of heat-killed *Lactobacillus paracasei* for treatment of perennial allergic rhinitis induced by house-dust mite. *Pediatric Allergy and Immunology* **16** (5) 433–438.

Prolo P, Chiappelli F, Fiorucci A, Dovio A, Sartori ML and Angeli A (2002) Psychoneuroimmunology: new avenues of research for the twenty-first century. *Annals of the New York Academy of Sciences* **966** 400–408.

Rachmilewitz D, Katakura K, Karmeli F, Hayashi T, Reinus C, Rudensky B, Akira S, Takeda K, Lee J, Takabayashi K and Raz E (2004) Toll-like receptor 9 signaling mediates the anti-inflammatory effects of probiotics in murine experimental colitis. *Gastroenterology* **126** (2) 520–528.

Roy-Byrne P (2006) A novel cytokine inhibitor effectively treats depression. *Journal Watch Psychiatry* **6**.

Rush AJ, Trivedi MH, Wisniewski SR, Nierenberg AA, Stewart JW, Warden D, Niederehe G, Thase ME, Lavori PW, Lebowitz BD, McGrath PJ, Rosenbaum JF, Sackeim HA, Kupfer DJ, Luther J and Fava M (2006) Acute and longer-term outcomes in depressed outpatients requiring one or several treatment steps: a STAR*D report. *American Journal of Psychiatry* **163** (11) 1905–1917.

Sakaguchi S (2004) Naturally arising CD4+ regulatory T cells for immunologic for self-tolerance and negative control of immune responses. *Annual Review of Immunology* **22** 531–562.

Shah A (1992) The burden of psychiatric disorder in primary care. *International Review of Psychiatry* **4** (3–4) 243–250.

Sharma MD, Baban B, Chandler P, Hou DY, Singh N, Yagita H, Azuma M, Blazar BR, Mellor AL and Munn DH (2007) Plasmacytoid dendritic cells from mouse tumor-draining lymph nodes directly activate mature Tregs via indoleamine 2,3-dioxygenase. *The Journal of Clinical Investigation* **117** (9) 2570–2582.

Silverman MN, Pearce BD, Biron CA and Miller AH (2005) Immune modulation of the hypothalamic- pituitary-adrenal (HPA) axis during viral infection. *Viral Immunology* **18** (1) 41–78.

Song C, Li X, Leonard BE and Horrobin DF (2003) Effects of dietary n-3 or n-6 fatty acids on interleukin-1beta-induced anxiety, stress, and inflammatory responses in rats. *Journal of Lipid Research* **44** (10) 1984–1991.

Suarez EC, Lewis JG and Kuhn C (2002) The relation of aggression, hostility, and anger to lipopolysaccharide-stimulated tumor necrosis factor (TNF)-alpha by blood monocytes from normal men. *Brain, Behavior, and Immunity* **16** 675–684.

Suarez EC, Lewis JG and Kuhn C (2004) Enhanced expression of cytokines and chemokines by blood monocytes to in vitro lipopolysaccharide stimulation are associated with hostility and severity of depressive symptoms in healthy women. *Psychoneuroendocrinology* **29** (9) 1119–1128.

Szabo S, Gould TD and Manji HK (2004) Neurotransmitters, receptors, signal transduction, and second messengers in psychiatric disorders. In: Schatzberg AF and Nemeroff CB (Eds) *Textbook of Psychopharmacology* (pp3–52). Arlington, VA: American Psychiatric Publishing.

Theoharides TC, Weinkauf C and Conti P (2004) Brain cytokines and neuropsychiatric disorders. *Journal of Clinical Psychopharmacology* **24** (6) 577–581.

Vollmer-Conna U, Fazou C, Cameron B, Li H, Brennan C, Luck L, Davenport T, Wakefield D, Hickie I and Lloyd A (2004) Production of pro-inflammatory cytokines correlates with the symptoms of acute sickness behaviour in humans. *Psychological Medicine* **34** (7) 1289–1297.

Wallace DJ (2001) Cytokines play an aetiopathogenetic role in fibromyalgia: a hypothesis and pilot study. *Rheumatology* (Oxford) **40** (7) 743–749.

Zhang L (2005) Alive and dead *Lactobacillus rhamnosus* GG decrease tumor necrosis factor-alpha-induced interleukin-8 production in Caco-2 cells. *Journal of Nutrition* **135** (7) 1752–1756.

Chapter 6
Omega-3 fatty acids for behaviour, learning and mood

DR ALEXANDRA J RICHARDSON

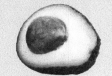

Increasing evidence suggests that relative deficiencies of EPA and DHA, the omega-3 fatty acids found in fish and seafood, may contribute not only to various physical illnesses (particularly cardiovascular and immune system disorders) but also to many disorders of mental health and performance across the lifespan (Peet *et al*, 2003; Bourre, 2004; Vaddadi, 2006).

Experts recommend a daily intake of at least 450–500 mg of EPA plus DHA for the general population simply to maintain cardiovascular health (Food and Behaviour Research, 2005) (achievable by eating two to four portions of fish per week), but average consumption in the UK and many other developed countries is less than half this level. Optimal intakes for brain function are not yet known, but the American Psychiatric Association (APA) recently reviewed the evidence for omega-3 in the prevention and treatment of psychiatric disorders (Freeman *et al*, 2006) and made the following recommendations:

■ all adults should eat fish at least twice a week
■ patients with mood, impulse control or psychotic disorders should consume one gram per day of EPA plus DHA
■ a supplement may be useful in patients with mood disorders (one to nine grams per day). Use of over three grams per day should be monitored by a physician.

It was emphasised that these recommendations are not a substitute for standard treatments for psychiatric disorders, as most trials to date have used omega-3 adjunctively.

Although folk wisdom has long held that 'fish is good for the brain', the mounting scientific evidence for this remains unfamiliar to many health professionals, who usually receive little or no training in nutrition. This chapter provides a summary overview of findings in this area to date, focusing on their practical implications.

Omega-3 and omega-6 fatty acids

Both omega-3 and omega-6 fatty acids are dietary essentials, but there are different forms of each and for optimal health, they need to be provided in the right balance. The two so-called 'essential fatty acids' (EFA) are alpha-linolenic acid (ALA) from the omega-3 series, and linoleic acid (LA) from the omega-6 series. These must come from the diet, as they cannot be manufactured within the body.

The forms of omega-3 and omega-6 that are most important for the brain, heart, immune system and other vital organs are not ALA and LA, however, but the more highly unsaturated fatty acids (HUFAs) – primarily DGLA and AA from the omega-6 series, and EPA and DHA from the omega-3 series, as shown in **Table 1**. In theory, these can be synthesised within the body from the respective EFA, but in practice, conversion is usually very limited, as discussed further below.

The so-called EFAs that cannot be synthesised within the body are LA (omega-6 series) and ALA (omega-3 series). The HUFAs that the brain needs can, in theory, be synthesised from these EFA precursors via processes of desaturation (insertion of a double-bond) and elongation (adding two carbon atoms to the fatty acid chain). However: *the conversion of EFAs to HUFAs is relatively slow and inefficient in humans*, so pre-formed HUFAs from dietary sources may be needed to ensure an adequate supply of these vital nutrients.

TABLE 1: PATHWAYS FOR THE SYNTHESIS OF OMEGA-6 AND OMEGA-3 FATTY ACIDS

Omega-6 series	Enzymes involved in **HUFA** synthesis	Omega-3 series
Linoleic (LA) 18:2		Alpha-linolenic (ALA) 18:3
|	*Delta 6-desaturase*	|
Gamma-linolenic 18:3		Octadecatetraenoic 18:4
|	*Elongase*	|
Dihomogamma-linolenic 20:3		Eicosatetraenoic 20:4
(DGLA)		|
|	*Delta 5-desaturase*	
Arachidonic (AA) 20:4		**Eicosapentaenoic (EPA) 20:5**
|	*Elongase*	|
Adrenic 22:4		Docosapentaenoic (DPA) 22:5
|	*Elongase, Delta 6-desaturase, Beta-oxidation*	|
Docosapentaenoic (DPA) 22:5		**Docosahexaenoic (DHA) 22:6**

Four HUFAs are particularly important for brain development and function: DGLA and AA from the omega-6 series, and EPA and DHA from the omega-3 series.

■ AA and DHA are major structural components of neuronal membranes (making up 20% of the dry mass of the brain and more than 30% of the retina).

■ EPA and DGLA are also crucial, but they play functional, rather than structural roles.

■ EPA, DGLA and AA are needed to manufacture eicosanoids – hormone-like substances including prostaglandins, leukotrienes, and thromboxanes. These and other HUFAs derivatives play critical roles in the moment-by-moment regulation of a very wide range of brain and body functions.

Fatty acids from one series cannot be converted into the other within the body. Both are essential, but the balance of omega-3 and omega-6 fatty acids is very important, as they play complementary roles in many biological functions, for example, derivatives of AA include the 'pro-inflammatory' series two prostaglandins, while DGLA and EPA give rise to less inflammatory prostaglandins (series one and series three respectively). Similarly, thromboxanes derived from AA act to constrict blood vessels while those derived from EPA act to relax blood vessels and improve blood flow.

Dietary sources of omega-3

Omega-6 fats are abundant in modern, Western-type diets. Vegetable oils (along with most nuts, seeds and grains) all tend to be rich in LA, such that this one substance now provides 8–10% of total calories in the average US diet. In addition, AA, the key omega-6 HUFA, is provided directly by meat, eggs and dairy produce.

By contrast, omega-3 fats are often relatively lacking, particularly from diets in which highly processed foods predominate. ALA is found in green, leafy vegetables and some nut and seed oils (notably flax and canola) as well as in seaweeds and algae, but fish and seafood are the only natural foods that provide appreciable quantities of the key omega-3 HUFAs EPA and DHA. Produce from grass-fed animals or wild game usually contain traces and food manufacturers are increasingly adding omega-3 to other products including milk, eggs and even bread, although these usually contain only small quantities.

Over the last century, ratios of omega-6 to omega-3 in Western-type diets have risen dramatically with increasing industrialisation of the food supply, from approximately 3:1 to more than 20:1 in some cases. This relative lack of omega-3 is thought to contribute to a wide range of both physical and mental health disorders (Simopoulos, 2002).

Omega-3 fatty acids and the brain

A huge research literature attests to the importance of omega-3 for healthy brain development and function. Both omega-3 and omega-6 HUFAs are essential to the brain, but, as already emphasised, omega-3 are the ones most likely to be lacking.

AA and DHA are both critical to the actual structure of all cell membranes in the brain and nervous system, making up 15% or more of the brain's dry mass, so adequate supplies are particularly important in early life. AA is crucial to brain and body growth and mild deficiencies during prenatal development are associated with low birth weight and reduced head circumference. DHA is particularly concentrated in highly active sites, such as synapses and photoreceptors, and makes up more than 30% of the retina, so this HUFA is vital for normal visual and cognitive development and function. Standard infant formula still contains only LA and ALA but increasing evidence shows that the addition of preformed AA and DHA (found naturally in breast milk) can be beneficial, particularly to premature infants (for an extremely comprehensive, open-access review of research in this area, see www.ahrq.gov/downloads/pub/evidence/pdf/o3maternalchild/o3mch.pdf).

During later childhood, and throughout life, a regular intake of HUFAs remains crucial to maintain the fluidity of neuronal membranes (which saturated fats and cholesterol act to reduce). Such fluidity is essential for optimal cell signalling, affecting the functioning of both neurotransmitter receptors and ion channels.

Concentrations of omega-3 and omega-6 HUFAs (and their balance) can also affect brain function in many other ways, on a moment-by-moment basis. Many chemical neurotransmitters, including dopamine and serotonin, can be influenced by HUFAs or their derivatives, as can numerous other biological processes, including programmed cell death, energy metabolism and gene expression.

The omega-3 EPA and the omega-6 DGLA and AA are all substrates for the eicosanoids, a highly bioactive group of hormone-like substances that includes prostaglandins, leukotrienes and thromboxanes, which help to regulate, among other things, hormonal, cardiovascular and immune systems. In terms of eicosanoid balance, the relative excess of AA (from meat, eggs and dairy products) relative to EPA (from fish and seafood) in typical Western diets will promote inflammation, enhance blood clotting and constrict blood vessels. It is easy to see how this could contribute to heart disease and inflammatory disorders, but the same signalling molecules can also exert profound influences on mental health and performance.

AA also gives rise to various 'endocannabinoids', which can influence mood, cognition and behaviour, as well as perception and sensitivity to pain, which have obvious relevance to many psychiatric disorders. Other important substances derived from either EPA or DHA can combat inflammation and/or help to protect brain cells against other types of injury (Serhan, 2005).

Why functional omega-3 HUFA deficiencies are common

Dietary deficiencies or imbalances of pre-formed HUFA

Most people in the UK and other developed countries fail to get from their diets the minimum 500 mg per day of EPA plus DHA recommended for heart health, but variations in background diet – particularly levels of the omega-6 LA and AA – mean that optimal intakes may actually be even higher. Using cross-national data these were estimated at 1,600 mg per day for the UK and 3,600 mg per day for the US to achieve tissue concentrations comparable to those of the Japanese, whose rates of physical and mental disorders associated with omega-3 deficiencies are among the world's lowest (Hibbeln *et al*, 2006).

Poor EFA–HUFA conversion

Vegetarians, vegans and others who don't eat fish, rely on the synthesis of EPA or DHA within the body. In general, this pathway is not efficient in humans, with estimated conversion rates from ALA of only around five per cent for EPA and less than one per cent for DHA (Brenna, 2002), but individual differences in this can reflect the following variable factors.

- **Normal genetic variation in the enzymes involved:** this genetic variation has recently been linked with individual variability in blood HUFA concentrations, the predisposition to ADHD and the effects of breastfeeding on children's IQ scores, although findings in each of these areas remain preliminary (details of these studies can be found at www.fabresearch.org).

- **Sex hormones and age:** efficiency of EFA–HUFA conversion is generally lower in males, young infants and the elderly and highest in women of childbearing age.

- **Diet and lifestyle factors:** synthesis of HUFAs from EFAs can be impaired by a dietary excess of saturated or hydrogenated fats, lack of vitamin and mineral co-factors (notably zinc, magnesium and vitamins A, B3, B6 and C) some viral infections and high levels of stress.

Smoking and/or excessive consumption of alcohol reliably depletes HUFA stores (rather than impairing synthesis), as can any other factors that increase oxidative stress, such as exposure to some environmental toxins and/or medications.

Other constitutional factors

Genetic variation in other aspects of fatty acid metabolism and/or antioxidant capacity may also affect an individual's dietary need for pre-formed HUFAs, but this remains an area of ongoing investigation.

Who is most likely to benefit from an increased dietary intake of omega-3 HUFA?

In the UK and US, pregnant mothers are currently advised to limit seafood consumption because of the theoretical risks of mercury and other possible neurotoxins. Recent evidence, however, indicates that this may actually be doing harm, and that higher seafood consumption during pregnancy leads to *better* motor skills, social and verbal abilities in children up to eight years of age, with no upper limit of benefit (Hibbeln *et al*, 2007).

Others who may benefit from increasing their omega-3 intake include:

- patients with depression, bipolar disorder or other psychiatric conditions, as recommended by the APA review of trials in this area (Freeman *et al*, 2006)

■ individuals with developmental conditions, including ADHD, dyslexia, dyspraxia and autistic spectrum disorders, although evidence from properly controlled trials is still limited (Richardson, 2006a)

■ older adults at risk of macular degeneration (a very common cause of loss of vision in the elderly) (Connor *et al*, 2007) or age-related cognitive decline. Several controlled trials are currently investigating omega-3 for this purpose in the general population. In the first study of Alzheimer's disease, benefits were found only for a subgroup of patients in the early stages (Freund-Levi *et al*, 2006).

The evidence that EPA and/or DHA may help in the management of adult psychiatric disorders appears strongest for conditions involving disturbances of mood/anxiety and/or impulse control. Since the APA review, benefits have been reported for patients with recurrent self-harm (Hallahan *et al*, 2007) and substance abusers (Buydens-Branchey and Branchey, 2006), and in major depression monotherapy with EPA yielding similar benefits to fluoxetine (Prozac), while the combination of both was superior to either treatment alone (Jazayeri *et al*, 2008). By contrast, trials with schizophrenia patients have shown mixed results for psychotic symptoms, but as the APA reviewers noted, an increased omega-3 intake could help to combat the increased risks of cardiovascular disease, diabetes and other physical health problems associated with schizophrenia, which some antipsychotic medications exacerbate.

In children, more large-scale studies are still needed, but results to date suggest that benefits from omega-3 supplementation may be greatest in those who have comorbid behaviour and learning difficulties (rather than those with 'pure' ADHD, dyslexia or similar diagnoses). Poor self-regulation of mood and attention may also help to predict treatment response, as discussed below. Some benefits for mood, impulsivity, stress-aggression and other aspects of behaviour or cognition have also been reported in psychiatrically normal populations (Hamazaki *et al*, 1996; Fontani *et al*, 2005).

It is most important to emphasise that dietary supplementation with omega-3 HUFAs cannot be expected to help all individuals with any particular diagnostic label, as the causes of these conditions are always complex and multi-factorial and will differ between individuals.

Clinically, blood biochemical measures of fatty acid status can be helpful if available, but these have their limitations, as discussed elsewhere (Richardson, 2006b). Otherwise, various features or symptoms that might help to predict a good response to an increased dietary intake of omega-3 HUFAs include the following (although each may have other causes).

■ Physical signs consistent with fatty acid deficiency such as excessive thirst, frequent urination, rough or dry skin and hair, dandruff, and soft or brittle nails and/or atopic tendencies (these could equally reflect deficiencies of the omega-6 GLA, found in evening primrose oil).

- Visual symptoms, particularly poor night vision, sensitivity to bright light (photophobia) and visual disturbances when reading.

- Attention and memory problems, including distractibility, difficulties with sustained concentration and working memory problems (often described as like 'brain fog'). These are typical of not only dyslexia, dyspraxia and ADHD, but also depression and age-related cognitive decline.

- Emotional sensitivity or instability, especially undue anxiety/tension, excessive mood swings, irritability or temper tantrums. Low frustration tolerance or 'short fuse syndrome' can underlie some of the impulsive, antisocial or otherwise inappropriate behaviours associated with ADHD, conduct disorder, oppositional defiant disorder, bipolar disorder and some personality disorders.

- Sleep problems, particularly difficulties in both falling asleep at night and waking up in the morning. There are numerous mechanisms by which omega-3 could affect general arousal and sleep–wake cycles (Yehuda, 2003).

Guidance for practitioners
Diet or supplements?
Like other nutrients, omega-3 is always best obtained from food if possible, but for those not willing or able to consume fish and seafood frequently, supplements are an obvious option.

Safety and tolerability
Up to three grams per day of EPA plus DHA from supplementation is generally regarded as a safe intake for the general population, but specialist supervision is likely to be advisable for regular supplementation of more than one gram per day, and always in consultation with medical or other professionals involved.

- Some types of fish and seafood carry possible contaminant risks and are best avoided by vulnerable groups, such as pregnant women or young children. As already noted, however, the benefits from consuming most types of seafood are likely to outweigh any such risks.

- The only known negative side effects of fish oil supplements are mild digestive symptoms, although these can often be minimised with the use of good quality supplements and/or attention to other aspects of the diet. In some cases, malabsorption may be an issue.

- High doses could interact with other medications, notably anticoagulants, which may, therefore, need to be monitored more regularly.

What formulation is optimal?

This will vary between individuals, in any case, and the evidence base from properly controlled trials in this area is too small to make definitive recommendations, but a few key issues are worth highlighting.

Omega-3: ALA versus EPA or DHA

Natural plant sources of omega-3 (such as flax oil) provide ALA, rather than EPA and DHA. This does not have the same health benefits and, as already emphasised, conversion within the body is very limited. For those seeking vegetarian options, DHA from algae is already available in supplement form (and is used in many infant formulae), but this did not appear to benefit children with ADHD or adults with depression in the only controlled trials to date (Richardson, 2008).

Omega-3: EPA versus DHA

As emphasised earlier, both EPA and DHA are essential to brain health, playing different but complementary roles. DHA is critical to the structure of cell membranes in the eyes, brain and nervous system, as well as the heart and other vital organs. EPA's role is more functional, as it gives rise to a wide range of regulatory substances that affect immune function, hormone balance and blood flow, among other things. Natural foods that provide EPA also provide DHA and any extremist claims for either one alone are likely to reflect commercial influences.

Standard fish oils usually have an EPA to DHA ratio of 3:2. Current evidence suggests that higher ratios than this may be more effective in improving mood and possibly other symptoms associated with developmental and psychiatric disorders (Fontani *et al*, 2005), although further research is still needed. Pure EPA has been used with success in several studies of adult psychiatric patients, but as conversion of EPA to DHA is limited (involving the same delta-6 desaturase enzymes that are rate-limiting at the initial step of EFA–HUFA conversion), the inclusion of at least some DHA may be helpful for many individuals. In pregnancy, early life and possibly in old age, higher ratios of DHA may be more appropriate but, again, this remains to be clarified by further research.

Is additional omega-6 needed?

Most people consume plenty of omega-6, but if EFA–HUFA conversion is poor, it is possible that DGLA levels might be compromised despite a high intake of LA and AA. GLA from evening primrose oil (EPO) could be helpful in such cases and controlled trials have shown this to be beneficial for atopic eczema and other skin conditions (Morse and Clough, 2006).

For behaviour, learning and mood, there is currently no good evidence that EPO alone is helpful, although supplements used in successful trials of omega-3 for child behaviour and learning to date have included some EPO (and vitamin E) (Richardson, 2006a) and anecdotal reports suggest that some such children may benefit from EPO in addition to fish oils.

Optimal dosages and monitoring response

Doses of 550–750 mg EPA plus DHA (in varying ratios) have shown benefits in controlled trials of children with dyslexia, dyspraxia and ADHD, but no dose-response studies have yet been carried out in this area. If behavioural problems and/or mood swings and impulsivity are severe, our clinical impressions suggest that one gram per day or more of EPA may be indicated, as recommended for depression and other mood disorders in adults.

Higher doses of pure EPA have shown benefits in some clinical trials of adult psychiatric disorders, but more is not always better, especially where individual nutrients are concerned. The only dose response studies to date indicate one gram per day of pure EPA as an optimal dose for depression (Peet and Horrobin, 2002) and two grams per day for schizophrenia (where any benefits were less clear in any case) (Peet *et al*, 2002), but doses of either one gram or two grams daily showed similar benefits over placebo in adults with bipolar disorder (Montgomery and Richardson, 2008).

Dietary HUFA requirements will differ between individuals and can also change in the same individual over time, so optimal dosages are best determined from careful monitoring, with attention paid to changes in any other factors that may be relevant.

Treatment duration and maintenance issues

Three months is the minimum recommended period for evaluating possible benefits from increasing omega-3 HUFA intake, as DHA concentrations in brain tissue can take this long to recover following chronic dietary deficiency. Having said this, clinical and research experience indicates that many people notice improvements on a much shorter timescale – usually within a week or two, and sometimes within days – and benefits seem to be lost just as quickly if supplementation is discontinued. The most notable subjective improvements usually involve better attention, concentration, mood and/or sleep.

Some commercial supplements state that daily intake can be reduced to a lower 'maintenance dose' after three months. Unfortunately, there remains no evidence to back these kinds of recommendations and our experience suggests that most people who derive any obvious benefits need to keep up an intake of around 500mg per day to maintain these. Furthermore, two studies that monitored children taking this kind of dose for up to six months indicate that some *additional* benefits may result from ongoing supplementation at this level.

Both dosage and maintenance issues need further research, but any dose changes should be as systematic as possible, with effects monitored for at least one to two weeks before further changes are instituted.

Other considerations

- Fish liver oils are not usually the best source of EPA and DHA for these purposes as large quantities could possibly lead to vitamin A toxicity in the long term. However, many UK children have inadequate intakes of vitamin A (and many other essential micronutrients), as discussed elsewhere (Richardson, 2006c) in which case, small quantities of fish liver oil could be useful. Anecdotal reports already suggest that some autistic children may benefit from small doses of cod liver oil and these merit proper investigation.

■ Quality of HUFA supplements is also crucial. EU regulations should ensure that fish oils contain no harmful residues, such as heavy metals, PCBs and dioxins, but these are not always well supervised and enforced by governments. Reputable suppliers should be able to provide evidence of good quality-control via independent testing.

■ HUFAs are particularly susceptible to oxidation if exposed to light, heat or air, and a good intake of vitamin E and other antioxidants including vitamin C is always advisable. Whole, unprocessed foods (particularly fruits, vegetables, nuts and seeds) are the best way to provide the full spectrum of antioxidants as well as other essential micronutrients. So, as always, the priority should be to achieve an overall balance to the diet.

Conclusions

Multiple strategies are usually needed for the optimal management of developmental and/or psychiatric disorders, and dietary interventions should always be complementary to other approaches. Optimising fatty acid intake is obviously only one aspect of good nutrition (albeit a central one), and there are many other dietary issues that should also be considered.

Omega-3 intake is widely acknowledged to be sub-optimal at the population level in the UK and most other developed countries, but some individuals may have unusually high dietary requirements for EPA and DHA while others need less than average. Given the evidence reviewed here, deficiencies are an obvious factor for practitioners to rule out when dealing with any patients who have difficulties in behaviour, learning or mood.

References

Bourre JM (2004) Roles of unsaturated fatty acids (especially omega-3 fatty acids) in the brain at various ages and during ageing. *Journal of Nutrition, Health and Aging* **8** (3) 163–174.

Brenna JT (2002) Efficiency of conversion of alpha-linolenic acid to long chain n-3 fatty acids in man. *Current Opinion in Clinical Nutrition and Metabolic Care* **5** (2) 127–132.

Buydens-Branchey L and Branchey M (2006) n-3 polyunsaturated fatty acids decrease anxiety feelings in a population of substance abusers. *Journal of Clinical Psychopharmacology* **26** (6) 661–665.

Connor KM, SanGiovanni JP, Lofqvist C, Aderman CM, Chen J, Higuchi A, Hong S, Pravda EA, Majchrzak S, Carper D, Hellstrom A, Kang JX, Chew EY, Salem N Jr, Serhan CN and Smith LEH (2007) Increased dietary intake of n-3 polyunsaturated fatty acids reduces pathological retinal angiogenesis. *Nature Medicine* **13** 868–873.

Fontani G, Corradeschi F, Felici A, Alfatti F, Migliorini S and Lodi L (2005) Cognitive and physiological effects of omega-3 polyunsaturated fatty acid supplementation in healthy subjects. *European Journal of Clinical Investigation* **35** (11) 691–699.

Food and Behaviour Research (2005) *Recommendations of the International Society for the Study of Fatty Acids and Lipids (ISSEAL) and the UK Joint Health Claims Initiative (JHCI)*. Further details can be found at the Food and Behaviour Research website: www.fabresearch.org.

Freeman MP, Hibbeln JR, Wisner KL, Davis JM, Mischoulon D, Peet M, Keck PE Jr, Marangell LB, Richardson AJ, Lake J and Stoll AL (2006) Omega-3 fatty acids: evidence basis for treatment and future research in psychiatry. *Journal of Clinical Psychiatry* **67** (12) 1954–1967.

Freund-Levi Y, Eriksdotter-Jonhagen M, Cederholm T, Basun H, Faxen-Irving G, Garlind A, Vedin I, Vessby B, Wahlund LO and Palmblad J (2006) Omega-3 fatty acid treatment in 174 patients with mild to moderate Alzheimer disease: OmegAD study: a randomized double-blind trial. *Archives of Neurology* **63** (10) 1402–1408.

Hallahan B, Hibbeln JR, Davis JM and Garland MR (2007) Omega-3 fatty acid supplementation in patients with recurrent self-harm: single-centre double-blind randomised controlled trial. *British Journal of Psychiatry* **190** (2) 118–122.

Hamazaki T, Sawazaki S, Itomura M, Asaoka E, Nagao Y, Nishimura N, Yazawa K, Kuwamori T and Kobayashi M (1996) The effect of docosahexaenoic acid on aggression in young adults. A placebo-controlled double-blind study. *Journal of Clinical Investigations* **97** (4) 1129–1133.

Hibbeln JR, Davis JM, Steer C, Emmett P, Rovers I, Williams C and Golding J (2007) Maternal seafood consumption in pregnancy and neurodevelopmental outcomes in childhood (ALSPAC study): an observational cohort study. *The Lancet* **369** (9561) 578–585.

Hibbeln JR, Nieminen LRG, Blasbalg TL, Riggs JA and Lands WEM (2006) Healthy intakes of n-3 and n-6 fatty acids: estimations considering worldwide diversity. *American Journal of Clinical Nutrition* **83** (suppl) 1483S–1493S.

Jazayeri S, Tehrani-Doost M, Keshavarz SA, Hosseini M, Djazayery A, Amini H, Jalali M and Peet M (2008) Comparison of therapeutic effects of omega-3 fatty acid eicosapentaenoic acid and fluoxetine, separately and in combination, in major depressive disorder. *Australian and New Zealand Journal of Psychiatry* **42** (3) 192–198.

Montgomery P and Richardson AJ (2008) Omega-3 fatty acids for bipolar disorder: a systematic review. *Cochrane Database of Systematic Reviews* **2**.

Morse NL and Clough PM (2006) A meta-analysis of randomized, placebo-controlled clinical trials of Efamol evening primrose oil in atopic eczema. Where do we go from here in light of more recent discoveries? *Current Pharmaceutical Biotechnology* **7** (6) 503–524.

Peet M, Glen I and Horrobin DF (Eds) (2003) *Phospholipid Spectrum Disorders in Psychiatry and Neurology.* Carnforth: Marius Press.

Peet M and Horrobin DF (2002) A dose-ranging study of the effects of ethyl-eicosapentaenoate in patients with ongoing depression despite apparently adequate treatment with standard drugs. *Archives of General Psychiatry* **59** (10) 913–919.

Peet M, Horrobin DF and E-E-Multicentre-Study-Group (2002) A dose-ranging exploratory study of the effects of ethyl-eicosapentaenoate in patients with persistent schizophrenic symptoms. *Journal of Psychiatry Research* **36** (1) 7–18.

Richardson AJ (2006a) Omega-3 fatty acids in ADHD and related neurodevelopmental disorders. *International Review of Psychiatry* **18** (2)155–172.

Richardson AJ (2006b) Omega-3 for child behaviour, learning and mood: ADHD, dyslexia, dyspraxia, autism and related conditions. *Nutrition Practitioner* (Summer).

Richardson AJ (2006c) *They Are What You Feed Them. How food can improve your child's behaviour, mood and learning.* London: HarperThorsons.

Richardson AJ (2008) Omega-3 fatty acids and mood: the devil is in the detail. *British Journal of Nutrition* **99** (2) 221–223.

Serhan CN (2005) Novel eicosanoid and docosanoid mediators: resolvins, docosatrienes, and neuroprotectins. *Current Opinion in Clinical Nutrition and Metabolic Care* **8** (2) 115–121.

Simopoulos AP (2002) The importance of the ratio of omega-6/omega-3 essential fatty acids. *Biomedicine and Pharmacotherapy* **56** (8) 365–379.

Vaddadi K (Ed) (2006) Essential fatty acids and mental illness. *International Review of Psychiatry* **18** (2) 81–186.

Yehuda S (2003) Omega-6/omega-3 ratio and brain-related functions. *World Review of Nutrition and Diet* **92** 37–56.

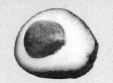

Chapter 7
Gut and psychology syndrome (GAP syndrome or GAPS)™

DR NATASHA CAMPBELL-MCBRIDE

We live in the world of unfolding epidemics. Autistic spectrum disorders, attention deficit hyperactivity disorder (ADHD/ADD), schizophrenia, dyslexia, dyspraxia, depression, obsessive-compulsive disorder, bipolar disorder and other neuro-psychological and psychiatric problems in children and adults are becoming more and more common (Papalos and Papalos, 2000; Ward, 2001; Holford, 2003; Shaw, 2002).

In clinical practice these conditions overlap with each other. A patient with autism is often hyperactive and dyspraxic. There is about 50% overlap between dyslexia and dyspraxia and 25–50% overlap between ADHD/ADD and dyslexia and dyspraxia (Holford, 2003; Shaw, 2002). Children with these conditions are often diagnosed as being depressed and as they grow up they are more prone to drug abuse or alcoholism than their typically developing peers (Holford, 2003; Shaw, 2002; Singh *et al*, 2001). A young person diagnosed with schizophrenia often suffered from dyslexia, dyspraxia and/or ADHD/ADD in childhood (Cade *et al*, 2000). When we start examining the patients with these so-called mental conditions, we find that they are also physically ill. Digestive problems, allergies, eczema, asthma, various food intolerances and immune system abnormalities are universally present among them (Singh *et al*, 2001; Cade *et al*, 2000; Dohan; 1969). We have created different diagnostic boxes for these patients, but a modern patient does not fit into any one of them neatly. The modern patient in most cases fits into a rather lumpy picture of overlapping neurological and psychiatric conditions.

Why are all these conditions related? What underlying problem are we missing?

To answer these questions we have to look at one factor that unites all these patients in a clinical setting. This factor is the state of their digestive system (Dohan *et al*, 1969; Dohan, 1969; Waring, 2001; Wakefield *et al*, 2000; Wakefield *et al*, 1998; Walker-Smith, 1998; Kawashima *et al*, 2000; Mycroft *et al*, 1982; Singh and Kay, 1976; Zioudrou *et al*, 1979; Baruk, 1978). I have yet to meet a child or an adult with autism, ADHD/ADD, dyspraxia, dyslexia, schizophrenia, bipolar disorder, depression or obsessive-compulsive disorder who does not have digestive abnormalities. In many cases they are severe enough for the patients or their parents to start talking about them first. In some cases the parents may not mention their child's digestive system, yet when asked direct questions, would describe a plethora of gut problems. So, what have digestive abnormalities got to do with these so-called mental problems? According to recent research and clinical experience, the answer is a lot. In fact, it appears that the patient's digestive system holds the key to the patient's mental state.

A typical scenario in clinical practice

Before examining the patient it is very important to look at the health history of the parents. Whenever the parents are mentioned, we immediately think about genetics. However, apart from genetics, there is something very important that the parents, in particular the mother, pass to their child: their unique gut micro-flora (Tabolin *et al*, 1998; Krasnogolovez, 1989; Lykova *et al*, 1999; Vorobiev *et al*, 1998). Not many people know that an adult carries, on average, two kilograms of bacteria in the gut. There are more cells in that microbial mass than there are cells in an entire human body (Krasnogolovez, 1989; Vorobiev *et al*, 1998). It is a highly organised micro world, where certain species of bacteria have to predominate to keep us physically and mentally healthy. Their role in our health is so monumental that we simply cannot afford to ignore them (Tabolin *et al*, 1998; Krasnogolovez, 1989; Lykova *et al*, 1999; Vorobiev *et al*, 1998). We will talk in detail about the child's gut flora later. Now let us come back to the source of the child's gut flora – the parents.

After studying hundreds of cases of neurological and psychiatric conditions in children and adults, a typical health picture of these children's mothers has emerged. An average modern mother typically was not breastfed as a baby, because she was born in the 1960s or 1970s when breastfeeding went out of fashion. This is important because it is now well-known that bottle-fed babies develop completely different gut flora to breastfed babies. This compromised gut flora in a bottle-fed baby predisposes it to many health problems later on. Having acquired compromised gut flora from the start, a typical modern mum has had quite a few courses of antibiotics in her childhood and youth for various infections. It is a well-known fact that antibiotics have a serious, damaging effect on gut flora, because they wipe out the beneficial strains of bacteria in the gut (Vorobiev *et al*, 1998; McCandless, 2003; Horvath *et al*, 1999). At the age of 16 (sometimes earlier), the modern mum was put on a contraceptive pill, which she took for quite a few years before starting a family. Contraceptive pills have a devastating effect on the beneficial (good) bacteria in the gut. One of the major functions of the good bacteria in the gut flora is to control about 500 different species of pathogenic (bad) and opportunistic microbes known to science. When the good bacteria are destroyed, the opportunists get a special opportunity to grow into large colonies and occupy large areas of the digestive tract. A modern diet of processed and fast food provides perfect nourishment for these pathogens and the typical diet that a modern mum had as a child and young adult would have included these foods. As a result of all these factors a modern mum has seriously compromised gut flora by the time she is ready to have children. Indeed, clinical signs of gut dysbiosis (abnormal gut flora) are present in almost 100% of mothers of children with neurological and psychiatric conditions (Vorobiev *et al*, 1998; McCandless, 2003; Horvath *et al*, 1999).

Why are we talking about mothers' gut flora? Because her baby is born with a sterile gut (Krasnogolovez, 1989; Lykova *et al*, 1999). In the first 20 or so days of life the baby's virgin gut surface is populated by a mixture of microbes. This is the gut flora, which will have a tremendous effect on this child's health for the rest of its life (Krasnogolovez, 1989; Lykova *et al*, 1999; Vorobiev *et al*, 1998). The gut flora mainly comes from the mother at the time of birth as she passes whatever microbial flora she has to her newborn child. Fathers with abnormal gut flora contribute to the bodily flora of the mother and through her to the gut flora of the child (Krasnogolovez, 1989; Lykova *et al*, 1999; Vorobiev *et al*, 1998; Lewis and Freedman, 1998).

The role and importance of the gut flora

Gut flora is something that we do not think about much. Yet, the number of functions that the gut flora fulfils are so vital for us that if our digestive tracts were sterilised, we probably would not survive (Krasnogolovez, 1989; Lykova *et al*, 1999; Vorobiev *et al*, 1998; Lewis and Freedman, 1998).

The first and very important function is *appropriate digestion and absorption of food*. If a child does not acquire normal balanced gut flora, then they will not digest and absorb foods properly, developing multiple nutritional deficiencies (Shaw, 2002; McCandless, 2003). This is what we commonly see in children and adults with learning disabilities, psychiatric problems and allergies. Many of these patients are malnourished. Even in the cases where the child may grow well, testing can reveal some typical nutritional deficiencies in many important minerals, vitamins, essential fats, many amino acids and other nutrients (Shaw, 2002; McCandless, 2003; Horvath *et al*, 1999; Schoenthaler *et al*, 1997). The most common deficiencies recorded in these patients are magnesium, zinc, selenium, copper, calcium, manganese, sulphur, phosphorus, iron, potassium, vanadium, boron, vitamins B1, B2, B3, B6, B12, C, A and D, folic acid, pantothenic acid, omegas -3, -6 and -9 fatty acids, taurine, alpha-ketoglutaric acid, glutathione and many other amino-acids. This usual list of nutritional deficiencies includes some most important nutrients for the normal development and functioning of the brain, immune system and rest of the body.

Apart from normal digestion and absorption of food, healthy *gut flora actively synthesises various nutrients*: vitamin K, pantothenic acid, folic acid, thiamine (vitamin B1), riboflavin (vitamin B2), niacin (vitamin B3), pyridoxine (vitamin B6), cyancobalamin (vitamin B12), various amino-acids and proteins. Indeed, when tested, people with gut dysbiosis present with deficiencies of these nutrients (Krasnogolovez, 1989; Vorobiev *et al*, 1998). Clinical experience shows that restoring the beneficial bacteria in their gut is the best way to deal with these deficiencies (Shaw, 2002; Krasnogolovez, 1989; Vorobiev *et al*, 1998; Lewis and Freedman, 1998).

The majority of children and adults with neurological and psychiatric conditions look pale and pasty. When tested, they show various stages of anaemia, which is not surprising (Krasnogolovez, 1989; Vorobiev *et al*, 1998; Lewis and Freedman, 1998). To have healthy blood we require many different nutrients: vitamins (B1, B2, B3, B6, B12, K, A, D, etc), minerals (iron, calcium, magnesium, zinc, cobalt, selenium, boron, etc), essential amino acids and fats. These patients not only can't absorb these nutrients from food, but their own production of many of them in the body is compromised (Krasnogolovez, 1989; Vorobiev *et al*, 1998; Lewis and Freedman, 1998). In addition, people with damaged gut flora often have particular groups of pathogenic bacteria growing in their gut, which are iron-loving bacteria (*Actinomyces* species, *Mycobacterium* species, pathogenic strains of *Escherichia coli*, *Corynebacterium* species and many others). These consume whatever iron the person gets from the diet, leaving them deficient in iron. Unfortunately, supplementing iron only supports these bacteria and does not remedy anaemia (Krasnogolovez, 1989). To treat anaemia, the person requires all the nutrients we have mentioned, many of which are supplied by healthy gut flora (Krasnogolovez, 1989; Vorobiev *et al*, 1998; Lewis and Freedman, 1998).

Apart from playing a vital part in nourishing the body, beneficial bacteria in the gut act as *the housekeepers for the digestive tract*. They coat the entire surface of the gut protecting it from invaders and toxins by providing a natural barrier and producing antibacterial, antiviral and antifungal substances (Krasnogolovez, 1989; Lykova *et al*, 1999; Vorobiev *et al*, 1998; Lewis and Freedman, 1998). At the same time they provide the gut lining with nourishment (Krasnogolovez, 1989). It is estimated that 60–70% of energy derived from the gut lining is from the activity of bacteria. Beneficial bacteria normally control various opportunistic and pathogenic microbes in the gut. Lack of beneficial bacteria would allow disease-causing microbes to grow and occupy large parts of the digestive system causing damage and inflammation in the gut wall (Krasnogolovez, 1989; Lykova *et al*, 1999; Vorobiev *et al*, 1998). Therefore, it is no surprise that when the gut flora is abnormal, the digestive tract itself cannot be healthy. Indeed, most patients with learning disabilities, psychiatric disorders and allergies present with digestive problems: constipation and diarrhoea, infantile colic and abdominal pain, bloating and flatulence, reflux and indigestion (Shaw, 2002; Baruk, 1978; Vorobiev *et al*, 1998; McCandless, 2003; Horvath *et al*, 1999). Examination by gastroenterologists commonly reveals inflammatory processes in the gut and many of these patients are diagnosed with coeliac disease (Wakefield *et al*, 2000; Wakefield *et al*, 1998; Walker-Smith, 1998; Mycroft *et al*, 1982; Singh and Kay, 1976; Zioudrou *et al*, 1979; Baruk, 1978; Dohan *et al*, 1984; Dohan, 1966). Housing a mass of pathogenic microbes in the gut cannot be healthy. Indeed, long before these patients develop so-called mental symptoms, they usually suffer from digestive problems and all other typical symptoms of gut dysbiosis, pretty much from the start of their lives (Shaw, 2002; Wakefield *et al*, 2000; Wakefield *et al*, 1998; Baruk, 1978; McCandless, 2003; Ashkenazi *et al*, 1979).

The role and importance of the immune system

A baby is born with an immature immune system (Kirjavainen *et al*, 1999). Establishment of healthy, balanced gut flora in the first few days of life plays a crucial role in appropriate maturation of the immune system (Krasnogolovez, 1989;

Lykova *et al*, 1999; Vorobiev *et al*, 1998). If the baby acquires compromised gut flora from the mother then it is left immune-compromised (Papalos and Papalos, 2000; Vorobiev *et al*, 1998; McCandless, 2003). The result is constant infections followed by courses of antibiotics, which damage the child's gut flora and immune system even further (Ward, 2001; Shaw, 2002; Vorobiev *et al*, 1998; Kirjavainen *et al*, 1999; Ferrari *et al*, 1988). The most common infections in the first two years of life in children with neurological, psychological and atopic disorders are ear infections, chest infections, sore throat and impetigo. Children also receive a lot of vaccinations in the first two years of life. A child with compromised immunity does not react to vaccinations in a predicted way. In many cases vaccines deepen the damage to the immune system and provide a source of chronic persistent viral infections and autoimmune problems in these children (Ward, 2001; Shaw, 2002; Vorobiev *et al*, 1998; Kirjavainen *et al*, 1999).

The good bacteria in the gut ensure appropriate production of different immune cells, immunoglobulins, keeping immunity in the right balance (Krasnogolovez, 1989; Lykova *et al*, 1999; Vorobiev *et al*, 1998). Damage inflicted on the gut flora typically leads to an imbalance between major parts of immunity, resulting in allergies, asthma and eczema – symptoms that children and adults with neurological and psychiatric conditions commonly suffer from (Kirjavainen *et al*, 1999; Lewis and Freedman, 1998; Ferrari *et al*, 1988; Ashkenazi *et al*, 1979).

There has been a considerable amount of research published on the state of the immune system in patients with learning disabilities and psychiatric problems (Shaw, 2002; Ferrari *et al*, 1988; Ashkenazi *et al*, 1979; Singh *et al*, 1988; Singh *et al*, 1991; Kontstantareas and Homatidis, 1987; Plioplys *et al*, 1994; Singh *et al*, 1998; Absolon *et al*, 1997; Furlano *et al*, 2001; Warren *et al*, 1986; Warren *et al*, 1987; Waizman *et al*, 1982; Yonk *et al*, 1990; Wakefield and Montgomery, 1999; Horrobin *et al*, 1994). The research shows deep abnormalities in all major cell groups and immunoglobulins. The most common autoantibodies found are to myelin basic protein (MBP) and neuron-axon filament protein (NAFP). These antibodies specifically attack the person's brain and the rest of the nervous system (Shaw, 2002; Singh *et al*, 1998; Warren *et al*, 1986; Waizman *et al*, 1982; Yonk *et al*, 1990; Horrobin *et al*, 1994).

Summary

A child with parents with abnormal gut flora has not acquired normal gut flora from the start (Shaw, 2002; Krasnogolovez, 1989; Lykova *et al*, 1999; Vorobiev *et al*, 1998; McCandless, 2003). The flora may have been damaged further by repeated courses of antibiotics and vaccinations (Ward, 2001; Krasnogolovez, 1989; Vorobiev *et al*, 1998; Samonis *et al*, 1994). As a result, these children commonly suffer from digestive problems, allergies, asthma and eczema (McCandless, 2003; Kirjavainen *et al*, 1999; Kontstantareas and Homatidis, 1987; Warren *et al*, 1986; Wakefield and Montgomery, 1999; Samonis *et al*, 1994; Rimland, 1994). However, in children and adults who go on to develop neurological and psychiatric problems, something even worse happens. Without control of the good bacteria, different opportunistic and pathogenic bacteria, viruses and fungi have a good chance to occupy large territories in the digestive tract. Two particular groups that are most commonly found on testing, are yeasts (including *Candida* species) and the clostridia family (Shaw, 2002; Baruk, 1978; Horrobin *et al*, 1994; Wilson *et al*, 1988; Samonis *et al*, 1994; Rimland, 1994; Bolte, 1998). These pathogenic microbes start digesting food in their own way, producing large amounts of various toxic substances, which are absorbed into the bloodstream, carried to the brain and cross the blood–brain barrier (Shaw, 2002; Lykova *et al*, 1999; Vorobiev *et al*, 1998; McCandless, 2003; Reichelt *et al*, 1981; Reichelt *et al*, 1990). The number and mixture of toxins can be very individual, causing different neurological and psychiatric symptoms. Due to the absence or greatly reduced numbers of beneficial bacteria in the gut flora, *the person's digestive system instead of being a source of nourishment, becomes a major source of toxicity in the body* (Ward, 2001; Shaw, 2002; Cade *et al*, 2000; Waring, 2001; Baruk, 1978; Krasnogolovez, 1989; Vorobiev *et al*, 1998; McCandless, 2003; Dohan *et al*, 1984; Absolon *et al*, 1997; Horrobin *et al*, 1994; Rimland, 1994).

What kind of toxic agents are there?

There are many toxins and we have not studied them in depth yet. However, some toxins have received a considerable amount of attention and are explained in more detail here.

Acetaldehyde and alcohol

The most common pathogenic microbes shown to overgrow in the digestive systems of children and adults with neuropsychiatric conditions are yeasts, particularly *Candida* species. Yeasts ferment dietary carbohydrates, producing alcohol and its by-product acetaldehyde. An overgrowth of yeast in the gut would constantly supply the body with these poisons flowing from the gut into the bloodstream. This condition was first described by Japanese researchers in the 1970s and 1980s and named an 'auto-brewery syndrome' (Shaw, 2002; Cade *et al*, 2000; Waring, 2001; Baruk, 1978; McCandless, 2003; Horrobin *et al*, 1994; Rimland, 1994). A constant exposure to alcohol and acetaldehyde has the following effects on the body:

■ liver damage with reduced ability to detoxify drugs, pollutants and other toxins.

■ pancreas degeneration with reduced ability to produce pancreatic enzymes, impairing digestion

■ reduced ability of the stomach wall to produce stomach acid

■ damage to immune system

■ brain damage with lack of self-control, impaired co-ordination, impaired speech development, aggression, mental retardation, loss of memory and stupor

■ peripheral nerve damage with altered senses and muscle weakness

■ direct muscle tissue damage with altered ability to contract and relax and muscle weakness

- nutritional deficiencies from damaging effects on digestion and absorption of most vitamins, minerals and amino acids – deficiencies in vitamins B and A are particularly common
- alcohol has an ability to enhance toxicity of most common drugs, pollutants and other toxins
- alteration of metabolism of proteins, carbohydrates and lipids in the body
- inability of the liver to dispose of old neurotransmitters, hormones and other by-products of normal metabolism; as a result these substances accumulate in the body, causing behavioural abnormalities and many other problems.

Acetaldehyde is considered to be the most toxic of alcohol by-products (Shaw, 2002; Cade *et al*, 2000; Baruk, 1978; Krasnogolovez, 1989; Absolon *et al*, 1997; Rimland, 1994). It is the chemical that gives us the feeling of a hangover. Anybody who has experienced a hangover knows how dreadful they felt. Children, who acquire abnormal gut flora with a lot of yeast from the start, may never know any other feeling. Acetaldehyde has a large variety of toxic influences on the body. One of the most devastating influences of this chemical is its ability to alter the structure of proteins, as altered proteins are thought to be responsible for many autoimmune reactions (Kirjavainen *et al*, 1999; Lewis and Freedman, 1998; Ferrari *et al*, 1988; Ashkenazi *et al*, 1979). Patients with neuropsychological problems are commonly found to have antibodies against their own tissues (Lewis and Freedman, 1998; Ferrari *et al*, 1988; Ashkenazi *et al*, 1979).

Clostridia neurotoxins

There are about 100 different clostridia species known so far (Shaw, 2002; Cade *et al*, 2000; Rimland *et al*, 1994). They are present in the faeces of people with autism, schizophrenia, psychosis, severe depression, muscle paralysis and muscle tone abnormalities and some other neurological and psychiatric conditions (Ward, 2001; Shaw, 2002; Cade *et al*, 2000; Waring; 2001; Baruk, 1978; Krasnogolovez, 1989; Vorobiev *et al*, 1998; McCandless, 2003; Dohan *et al*, 1984; Absolon *et al*, 1997; Horrobin *et al*, 1994; Rimland, 1994). Many clostridia species are normal inhabitants of the human gut. *Clostridium tetani*, for example, is routinely found in the gut of healthy humans and animals. However, it can produce an extremely powerful neurotoxin that causes the deadly disease, tetanus. *Clostridium tetani*, which lives in the gut, is normally controlled by the beneficial bacteria and does us no harm, because its toxin cannot get through the healthy gut wall.

Patients with disturbed gut flora do not have a healthy gut wall and these powerful neurotoxins are absorbed through the damaged gut lining, then cross the blood–brain barrier, affecting the patient's mental functioning (Ward, 2001; Shaw, 2002; Vorobiev *et al*, 1998; McCandless, 2003; Horrobin *et al*, 1994; Rimland, 1994). Many other species of clostridia (perfringens, novyi, septicum, histolyticum, sordelli, aerofoetidum, tertium, sporogenes) produce toxins similar to tetanus toxin, as well as many others. William Shaw at Great Plains Laboratories describes in detail a number of autistic children who showed considerable improvements in their development and biochemical tests while on anticlostridia medication (2002). However, as soon as the medication was stopped, the children slipped back into autism as they did not have a healthy gut flora to control clostridia. In many cases clostridia is not identified in the faeces of these children because it is strictly anaerobic and very difficult to study. Professor Gibson of Reading University in the UK has identified clostridia overgrowth in the gut of autistic children and his team is working on finding effective treatments for the problem (Ward, 2001; Shaw, 2002; McCandless, 2003; Dohan *et al*, 1984; Rimland, 1994).

Yeasts and clostridia have been given a special opportunity during the era of antibiotics. Broad-spectrum antibiotics do not touch them, but eliminate the good bacteria in the gut, which normally control yeasts and clostridia. The patients we are talking about are usually exposed to numerous courses of antibiotics early in their lives.

Gluteomorphins and casomorphins (opiates from gluten and casein)

Opiates are drugs – like opium, morphine and heroin – that are commonly used by drug addicts. What have they got to do with our patients?

Gluten is a protein present in grains, mainly wheat, rye, oats and barley. Casein is a milk protein, present in cow, goat, sheep, human and all other animal milk and milk products. In gut dysbiosis these proteins do not have a chance to be digested properly before they are absorbed in the form of substances with a similar chemical structure to opiates, like morphine and heroin. There has been quite a substantial amount of research done in this area by Dohan, Reichelt, Shattock, Cade and others, where gluten and casein peptides, called gluteomorphins and casomorphins, were detected in the urine of schizophrenic patients, autistic and ADHD children and patients with depression and autoimmune conditions (Ward, 2001; Shaw, 2002; Cade *et al*, 2000; Waring; 2001; Baruk, 1978; Krasnogolovez, 1989; Vorobiev *et al*, 1998; McCandless, 2003; Dohan *et al*, 1984; Singh *et al*, 1998; Horrobin *et al*, 1994; Rimland, 1994). These opiates from wheat and milk enter the blood–brain barrier and block certain areas of the brain, just like morphine or heroin, causing various neurological and psychological symptoms.

We have mentioned a few toxins found in these patients. There are many others currently being studied. The mixture of toxicity in each child or adult can be quite individual and different. But what they all have in common is gut dysbiosis (abnormal gut flora). The toxicity, which is produced by the abnormal microbial mass in these patients, establishes a link between the gut and the brain. That is why it is logical to group these disorders under one name: gut and psychology syndrome (GAPS)™. GAPS children and adults can present with symptoms of autism, ADHD, ADD, OCD, dyslexia, dyspraxia, schizophrenia, depression, bipolar disorder, sleep disorders, allergies, asthma and eczema in any possible combination. These are the patients who fall through the gap in our medical knowledge. Any child or adult with a learning disability, neurological or psychological problems and allergies should be thoroughly examined for gut dysbiosis. Re-establishing normal gut flora and treating the digestive system of the person has to be the number one priority for these disorders, before considering any other treatments with drugs or otherwise (Krasnogolovez, 1989; Lykova *et al*, 1999; Vorobiev *et al*, 1998; McCandless, 2003; Schoenthaler *et al*, 1997; Lewis and Freedman, 1998; Macfarlane and Cummings, 1999; Ward, 1997).

GAPS establishes the connection between the state of the patient's gut and the functioning of the brain. This connection has been known by medics for a very long time. The father of modern psychiatry French Psychiatrist Phillipe Pinel (1745–1828), after working with mental patients for many years, concluded in 1807: *'The primary seat of insanity generally is in the region of the stomach and intestines'* (Horrobin *et al*, 1994). Long before him, Hippocrates (460–370 BC), the father of modern medicine, said: *'All diseases begin in the gut!'* (Krasnogolovez, 1989; Lykova *et al*, 1999; Vorobiev *et al*, 1998). The more we learn with our modern scientific tools, the more we realise just how right they were.

In order to help patients with GAPS, we have to concentrate on treating the patient's digestive system: we need to re-establish normal gut flora and heal and seal the damaged gut lining. Healing the digestive system stops the flow of toxins from the gut to the brain and as a result removes or reduces the plethora of mental and neurological symptoms that the patient displays (Papalos and Papalos, 2000; Holford, 2003; Shaw, 2002; Dohan *et al*, 1969; Dohan, 1969; Mycroft *et al*, 1982; Singh and Kay, 1976; Baruk, 1978). As the gut starts functioning normally, the food is digested and absorbed properly. As a result, the patient becomes healthier physically as well as mentally. All this can be achieved with the GAPS Nutritional Protocol, consisting of a very specific diet, nutritional supplementation and some changes in the lifestyle of the patient. How GAPS develops and how to treat it effectively with a sound nutritional protocol cannot be described in detail here. Interested readers should refer to my book, *Gut and Psychology Syndrome. Natural treatment for autism, ADHD/ADD, dyslexia, dyspraxia, depression and schizophrenia*. This programme has been used by thousands of patients in recent years with good results: patients diagnosed with autism, dyslexia, dyspraxia, ADHD/ADD, schizophrenia, bipolar disorder, depression, epilepsy and other so-called mental and neurological conditions.

References

Absolon CM, Cottrell D, Eldridge SM and Glover MT (1997) Psychological disturbance in atopic eczema: the extent of the problem in school-aged children. *British Journal of Dermatology* **137** (2) 241–245.

Ashkenazi A, Krasilowsky D, Levin S, Idar D, Kalian M, Or A, Ginat Y and Halperin B (1979) Immunologic reaction in psychotic patients to fractions of gluten. *American Journal of Psychiatry* **136** (10) 1306–1309.

Baruk H (1978) Psychoses of digestive origins. In: G Hemmings and WA Hemmings (Eds) *Biological Basis of Schizophrenia*. Lancaster: MTP Press.

Bolte ER (1998) Autism and *Clostridium tetani*. *Medical Hypothesis* **51** (2) 133–144.

Cade RJ, Privette RM, Fregly M, Rowland N, Sun Z, Zele V, Wagemaker H, Edelstrein C (2000) Autism and schizophrenia: intestinal disorders. *Nutritional Neuroscience* **2** 57–72.

Dohan FC (1966) Cereals and schizophrenia: data and hypothesis. *Acta Psychiatrica Scandinavica* **42** (2) 125–152.

Dohan FC (1969) Is celiac disease a clue to pathogenesis of schizophrenia? *Mental Hygiene* **53** (4) 525–529.

Dohan FC, Grasberger JC, Lowell FM, Johnston HT Jr and Arbegast AW (1969) Relapsed schizophrenics: more rapid improvement on a milk and cereal free diet. *British Journal of Psychiatry* **115** (522) 595–596.

Dohan FC, Harper EH, Clark MH, Rodrigue RB and Zigas V (1984) Is schizophrenia rare if grain is rare? *Biology and Psychiatry* **19** (3) 385–399.

Ferrari P, Marescot M, Moulias R, Bursztejn C, Deville-Chambrolle A, Thiolett M, Lesourd B, Braconnier A, Dreux C and Zarifian E (1988) Immune status in infantile autism: correlation between the immune status, autistic symptoms and levels of serotonin. *L'Encephale* **14** (5) 339–344.

Furlano RI, Anthony A, Day R, Brown A, McGarvey L, Thomson MA, Davies SE, Berelowitz M, Forbes A, Wakefield AJ, Walker-Smith JA and Murch SH (2001) Colonic CD8 and gamma delta T-cell infiltration with epithelial damage in children with autism. *The Journal of Pediatrics* **138** (3) 366–372.

Holford P (2003) *Optimum Nutrition for the Mind*. London: Piatkus.

Horrobin DF, Glen AM and Vaddadi K (1994) The membrane hypothesis of schizophrenia. *Schizophrenia Research* **18** 195–207.

Horvath K, Papadimitriou JC, Rabsztyn A, Drachenberg C and Tildon JT (1999) Gastrointestinal abnormalities in children with autism. *Journal of Pediatrics* **135** 559–563.

Kawashima H, Takayuki M, Kashiwagi Y, Takekuma K, Hoshika A and Wakefield AJ (2000) Detection and sequencing of measles virus from peripheral blood mononuclear cells from patients with inflammatory bowel disease and autism. *Digestive Diseases and Sciences* **45** (4) 723–729.

Kirjavainen PV, Apostolov E, Salminen SS and Isolauri E (1999) New aspects of probiotics – a novel approach in the management of food allergy. *Allergy* **54** (9) 909–915.

Kontstantareas M and Homatidis S (1987) Ear infections in autistic and normal children. *Journal of Autism and Developmental Disorders* **17** (4) 585–593.

Krasnogolovez VN (1989) *Colonic Disbacteriosis* (Russian). Moscow: Medicina.

Lewis SJ and Freedman AR (1998) Review article: the use of biotherapeutic agents in the prevention and treatment of gastrointestinal disease. *Alimentary Pharmacology and Therapeutics* **12** (9) 807–822.

Lykova EA, Bondarenko VM, Sidorenko SV, Grishina ME, Murashova AD, Minaev VI, Rytikov FM and Korsunski AA (1999) Combined antibacterial and probiotic therapy of Helicobacter – associated disease in children (Russian). *Zhurnal Microbiologii, Epidemiologii I Immunobiologii* **2** (Mar–Apr) 76–81.

Macfarlane GT and Cummings JH (1999) Probiotics and prebiotics: can regulating the activities of intestinal bacteria benefit health? (Review) *British Medical Journal* **318** (7189) 999–1003.

McCandless J (2003) *Children with Starving Brains.* Paterson, NJ: Bramble Books.

Mycroft FJ, Wei ET, Bernardin JE and Kasarda DD (1982) JIF-like sequences in milk and wheat proteins. *New England Journal of Medicine* **307** (14) 895.

Papalos D and Papalos J (2000) *The Bipolar Child.* New York: Broadway Books.

Plioplys AV, Greaves A, Kazemi K and Silverman E (1994) Lymphocyte function in autism and Rett syndrome. *Neuropsychobiology* **7** (1) 12–16.

Reichelt KL, Ekrem J and Scott H (1990) Gluten, milk proteins and autism: dietary intervention effects on behaviour and peptide secretions. *Journal of Applied Nutrition* **42** 1–11.

Reichelt KL, Hole K, Hamberger A, Saelid G, Edminson PD, Braestrup CB, Lingjaerde O, Ledaal P and Orbeck H (1981) Biologically active peptide-containing fractions in schizophrenia and childhood autism. *Advances in Biochemical Psychopharmacology* **28** 627–647.

Rimland B (1994) New hope for safe and effective treatments for autism. *Autism Research Review International* **8** (3).

Samonis G, Gikas A and Toloudis P (1994) Prospective evaluation of the impact of broad-spectrum antibiotics on the yeast flora of the human gut. *European Journal of Clinical Microbiology and Infections Diseases* **13** (8) 665–657.

Schoenthaler S, Amos S, Doraz W, Kelly M, Muedeking G and Wakefield J (1997) The effect of randomised vitamin-mineral supplementation on violent and non-violent antisocial behaviour among incarcerated juveniles. *Journal of Nutritional and Environmental Medicine* **7** (4) 343–352.

Shaw W (2002) *Biological Treatments for Autism and PDD.* Lenexa: The Great Plains Laboratory.

Singh MM and Kay SR (1976) Wheat gluten as a pathogenic factor in schizophrenia. *Science* **191** (4225) 401–402.

Singh V (1988) Immunodiagnosis and immunotherapy in autistic children. *Annals of the New York Academy of Sciences* **540** 602–604.

Singh V, Fudenberg HH, Emerson D and Coleman M (2001) Neuro-immunopathogenesis in autism. In: I Berczi and RM Gorczynski (Eds) *New Foundations of Biology* (pp447–458). Amsterdam: Elsevier Science.

Singh V, Warren RP, Odell JD and Cole P (1991) Changes in soluble interleukin-2, interleukin-2 rector, T8 antigen, and interleukin-I in the serum of autistic children. *Clinical Immunology and Immunopathology* **61** (3) 448–455.

Singh VK, Lin SX and Yang VC (1998) Serological association of measles virus and human herpesvirus-6 with brain autoantibodies in autism. *Clinical Immunology and Immunopathology* **89** (1) 105–108.

Tabolin VA, Belmer SV, Gasilina TV, Muhina UG and Korneva TI (1998) *Rational Therapy of Intestinal Dysbacteriosis in Children* (Russian). Moscow: Medicina.

Vorobiev AA, Pak SG, Savizkaja KE, Bondarenko VM, Nesvizencki UV, Malov VA, Likova EA, Mazulevich TV, Abramov NA, Murashova AO, Trofimenko LS, Minaev VA and Sherbakov PL (1998) *Dysbacteriosis in Children* (Russian). Moscow: KMK Lt.

Waizman A, Weizman R, Szekely GA, Wijsenbeek H and Livni E (1982) Abnormal immune response to brain tissue antigen in the syndrome of autism. *American Journal of Psychiatry* **139** (11) 1462–1465.

Wakefield AJ, Anthony A, Murch SH, Thomson M, Montgomery SM, Davies S, O'Leary JJ, Berelowitz M and Walker-Smith JA (2000) Enterocolitis in children with developmental disorders. *American Journal of Gastroenterology* **95** (9) 2285–2295.

Wakefield AJ and Montgomery SM (1999) Autism, viral infection and measles, mumps, rubella vaccination. *Israeli Medical Association Journal* **1** (November) 183–187.

Wakefield AJ, Murch SH, Anthony A, Linnell J, Casson DM, Malik M, Berelowitz M, Dhillon AP, Thomson MA, Harvey P, Valentine A, Davies SE and Walker-Smith JA (1998) Ileal-lymphoid-nodular hyperplasia, non-specific colitis and pervasive developmental disorder in children. *The Lancet* **351** (9103) 637–641.

Walker-Smith JA (1998) Autism, inflammatory bowel disease and MMR vaccine. *The Lancet* **351** (9106) 1356–1357.

Ward NI (1997) Assessment of clinical factors in relation to child hyperactivity. *Journal of Nutritional and Environmental Medicine* **7** (4) 333–342.

Ward NI (2001) Hyperactivity and a previous history of antibiotic usage. *Nutrition Practitioner* **3** (3) 12.

Waring (2001) *Sulphate, Sulphation and Gut Permeability: Are cytokines involved?* Conference proceedings at The Biology of Autism – Unravelled, 11 May 2001. London: Institute of Electrical Engineers.

Warren RP, Foster A and Margaretten NC (1987) Reduced natural killer cell activity in autism. *Journal of the American Academy of Child Psychiatry* **26** (3) 333–335.

Warren RP, Margaretten NC, Pace NC and Foster A (1986) Immune abnormalities in patients with autism. *Journal of Autism and Developmental Disorders* **16** 189–197.

Wilson K, Moore L, Patel M and Permoad P (1988) Suppression of potential pathogens by a defined colonic microflora. *Microbial Ecology in Health and Disease* **1** (4) 237–243.

Yonk LJ, Warren RP, Burger RA, Cole P, Odell JD, Warren WL, White E and Singh VK (1990) D4+ per T cell depression in autism. *Immunology Letters* **35** (4) 341–346.

Zioudrou C, Streaty RA and Klee WA (1979) Opioid peptides derived from food proteins. The exorphins. *The Journal of Biological Chemistry* **254** 2446–2449.

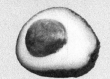

Chapter 8

Duncan's story: a case history of institutional discrimination in the NHS

LINDA TROTT AND LAURIE TROTT

Laurie

In this chapter, we will describe the experience of one young man in the mental health system in the UK. The chapter will illustrate how institutional discrimination occurs against those with nutritional and other health issues. I will first offer a definition and understanding of what constitutes institutional discrimination then my wife, Linda, will describe the experience and treatment of my stepson, Duncan, in the mental health system. We intend that you will clearly see how he was discriminated against, not only in terms of his nutritional needs, but in other ways as well.

First, it is necessary to develop an understanding of institutional discrimination. In modern times, the Stephen Lawrence Inquiry gave us an understanding of institutional *racism*, but the concept and, indeed, the practice of institutional discrimination has been around for centuries. It is useful however, to look at the definition of institutional racism according to McPherson (1999) in the Lawrence Inquiry report and extrapolate this into a more general understanding of institutional discrimination. According to McPherson:

> 'Institutional racism [discrimination] *consists of the collective failure of an organisation to provide an appropriate and professional service to people because of their colour, culture or ethnic origin* [social or biological difference]. *It can be seen or detected in processes, attitudes and behaviour which amount to discrimination through unwitting prejudice, ignorance, thoughtlessness and racist stereotyping which disadvantage minority ethnic* [these] *groups.'*

The bracketed words are my alternatives to the words preceding them and convert this definition of institutional racism into a more general definition of institutional discrimination.

The strength of the McPherson definition is that it highlights a critical aspect of institutional discrimination – this being the *collective failure* of organisations to account for difference. Therefore, institutional discrimination most often consists not of actions but inactions. To put this another way, it is what organisations *fail* to do when faced with any individual or group that is not best served by its existing policies, procedures and practices or whose needs fall outside of their normal operating parameters.

Second, institutional discrimination is most often *unconscious* on the part of individuals within the organisation. If such actions were made consciously, it is likely that at some stage someone in the organisation would challenge and change them. Finally, it is important to note that McPherson also highlights the fact that it can be detected by the ignorance of the individuals practising the discrimination. Usually this ignorance consists of another failure: to consider that the paradigm in which they operate may be flawed or incomplete. As we will see from this case study, mental health services are permeated with institutional discrimination typified by unconscious inaction, ignorance and failures.

Linda

Duncan was born in 1985. He had a normal birth and was a thriving child. When he started to eat solid food, he became increasingly ill. He began to projectile vomit after eating and to lose weight dramatically. Following extensive testing, Duncan was finally sent to a London hospital to see an allergist. It was found that he had allergies to many foods, including wheat, artificial colourants and additives. I put him on a restricted diet, which excluded all additives and foods that he was sensitive to. Following this regime, Duncan improved dramatically, regaining weight and full health… or so I thought.

When he was 14 months old he developed a high temperature and a red rash and was admitted into the isolation unit of the local hospital. A diagnosis of severe roseola infection was made.

When Duncan was around two years old he became hyperactive, unable to sleep or to concentrate. I contacted Sally Bunday, Director of the Hyperactive Children's Support Group. She recommended the Feingold Diet and supplementation with omega oils and nutrients such as zinc and vitamin B6. By readjusting his diet and taking supplements, we were able to restore his health once again.

At the age of 10, Duncan began to have difficulties in school. The diagnosis was dyslexia and he joined a special needs group. Once again, I researched this condition and found a supplement containing high quantities of omega-3 oil. After three months at maximum dosage Duncan was able to rejoin his peers in mainstream classes and within a year he was an above-average pupil in reading. He continued to take a maintenance dose of omega-3.

At the age of 15, Duncan and some friends smoked cannabis. While his friends could cope with the effects of the drug, Duncan became dramatically ill. He lost a considerable amount of weight, was physically exhausted and slept most of the time. He became agoraphobic and showed signs of paranoia. However, he did not have delusions or hallucinations and did not hear voices.

In July 2002, after several weeks of illness and on the advice of his GP, Duncan was voluntarily admitted to hospital (the only child on an adult ward). He was still smoking cannabis at this time. The Consultant Psychiatrist told us that he was *probably self-medicating*. He was tested for cannabis and found positive.

When admitted into hospital he was immediately put on three drugs:

- 10 mg olanzapine daily
- 20 mg citalopram daily
- 50 mg chlorpromazine at night.

At no time was he given any physical examination or clinical tests. I told the psychiatric team of Duncan's medical history and nutritional needs, but these were dismissed as irrelevant by the psychiatrist (Dr M). I was not allowed to give Duncan any nutritional supplements on the ward, even though I made several requests to do so.

We found out by accident that he had been diagnosed with schizophrenia, despite Duncan not displaying most of the symptoms of this condition. When asked for a prognosis, we were callously given one word: 'poor'. On this mixture of prescribed drugs Duncan developed disturbing symptoms, including a racing pulse, pounding heart and excessive sweating. When he got up from a sitting or lying position he would complain of feeling faint and dizzy. He started to have a voracious appetite and an inability to focus his gaze. He was unable to communicate and was almost monosyllabic. His paranoia did not abate and he was still agoraphobic, although testing negative for cannabis. He started to have panic attacks.

By now, Duncan had put on a large amount of weight (two stone in six weeks). Such was my concern that I wrote a comprehensive medical history of Duncan and his family and gave copies to Dr M and other psychiatric staff at ward round. I told everyone present of my deep concern at Duncan's new symptoms and asked for a reduction of the drugs. Having researched all three of these drugs, I knew that there had been no clinical trials using them in combination. Most disturbingly, olanzapine was not recommended for children under 18 years old and, in common with all such drugs, had never been tested on children. I was particularly concerned about olanzapine as this is contra-indicated where there is a history of familial diabetes (Duncan's father has diabetes). I also made it clear that I believed Duncan needed nutritional supplements to stay healthy. I tried to give out copies of my research but the response of the psychiatric team was either silence or disdainful looks.

I was so concerned at the complete disinterest of the medical team in Duncan's declining health that I contacted the Schizophrenia Association of Great Britain (SAGB). I spoke to Gwyneth Hemmings (Director) and Dr Yung Wei (Research Scientist). I took Duncan from the hospital to the SAGB in Bangor and had his blood tested after fasting him for 12 hours.

Dr Yung Wei shared his extensive research on the connection between coeliac disease and schizophrenic symptoms. His research showed that anyone with a history of wheat allergy was most likely to be genetically disposed to present symptoms of mental illness under certain conditions. He advised that a complete physical examination should take place (as well as blood tests) on all patients in Duncan's position as it is imperative to ensure that there are no underlying physical conditions that could lead to a misdiagnosis of schizophrenia. He advised me to give Duncan omega-3 oil to displace the raised triglycerides.

The results of the blood test showed that Duncan's triglyceride level was twice the upper range of normal. This was very disturbing, given Duncan's family history of diabetes and heart attacks. I sent a letter to Dr M detailing the results of the blood test and another copy of the family history. When I spoke to Dr M about this result, he stated that the result was so high because Duncan had not fasted for 12 hours – although as I had been with Duncan and Dr M hadn't, I'm not sure how he could have known this! As a result of sending the letter, Duncan was sent for a further triglyceride test as Dr M did not accept the previous result. The test results confirmed that his triglyceride levels were very high. These results, together with other important medical notes, mysteriously went missing some time later and were never shown to me. A week later, a member of the medical team told me that Dr M had sent every other patient in the hospital who was taking olanzapine for a triglyceride test.

At the next ward round I asked for Duncan to be allowed to take omega-3. Another doctor (Dr D) asked me if I really believed that I could improve Duncan's condition with fish oils and vitamins. I attempted to explain that I had already improved his mental function with such treatment. Dr D simply stared at me and then two other team members of the medical team simply shook their heads and smiled. As a result of this, I started to smuggle Duncan's supplements onto the ward.

I gave Dr M research from the SAGB, plus my own research about the warnings that olanzapine causes problems with blood–sugar levels in young patients and, in some cases, early onset diabetes, as well as information on how omega-3 and other supplements can improve mental function. I again stated my concern at Duncan's huge weight gain. Dr M then asked me if there was any family history of diabetes. I pointed out that I had stated this three times, twice in writing and once verbally and that the letters I had written to this effect were in front of him in the folder.

Duncan was discharged from hospital in October, still displaying all of the symptoms above. The medication of olanzapine continued. He was continually hungry, craved tobacco and was exhausted all the time. He was unable to function normally.

The results of private cytotoxic blood tests that we had carried out that month showed that Duncan had intolerances to a plethora of foods (especially wheat), additives and colourants. He was also suffering from gut dysbiosis due to yeast overgrowth in the gut, and multiple vitamin and mineral deficiencies. It was advised that Duncan remove wheat and milk from his diet immediately, as he is intolerant to them and there is evidence to support that both can cause cerebral allergy and psychosis.

Duncan's health began to decline in January 2003 and he was readmitted to hospital that month. We asked Dr M if we could give Duncan nutritional supplements and if a wheat- and dairy-free diet could be provided. Their attitude was dismissive and sometimes even hostile. Dr M and other staff eventually said that they *'would try'* to obtain a suitable diet. Eventually, I persuaded the nurses to allow me to bring bags containing daily doses of omega-3 and other nutrients that I had prepared, which would be offered to Duncan.

By the end of May 2003 Duncan was continuing to gain weight alarmingly. Despite his allergy to wheat, all that was available to him and all other patients for the evening meal were pre-packed sandwiches. I invited Dr M to contact the nutritionist advising Duncan (Frank McGowan) and was told by Dr M that: *'I do not need to speak to him but if he wants to speak to my nurses that's up to them.'*

Duncan was offered a place in Progress House (PH), a home where people recovering from mental illness could progress to integrate into the community. He moved there shortly afterwards. In July 2003 I attended a progress review in PH with Duncan. The attending Psychiatrist (Dr S) asked me why Duncan was following an exclusion diet. I explained the reasons. Dr S said that in her view he would become malnourished if he didn't eat things like tomatoes (despite Duncan being 6 foot 3 inches and well built!) and said in a hostile and dismissive manner: *'Well if you insist on this, I suppose we'll have to go along with it.'*

In September 2003 a new Psychiatrist (Dr P) took over as Duncan's consultant. (Dr M went on extended leave and never came back.) A meeting took place in September between the medical staff in charge of Duncan, my husband and I. I presented all the findings from private tests of the last six months. As a result of this, Dr P agreed that there *could be* some foundation to the findings that Duncan was suffering from a physical illness. He agreed to liaise with a Nutritionist who was also medically qualified (Dr Campbell McBride) and, in addition, with any other medical practitioner that might be able to help.

In October 2003 I attended a consultation with Dr Campbell-McBride. She made many recommendations as to diet and treatment, which Dr P accepted *'might have some merit'* and, as she was an expert in the field, he agreed to support Dr Campbell-McBride's recommendations.

After a few months Duncan had improved a little and was considered well enough to move to a supported flat, which he did in 2005. However, his condition deteriorated for no apparent reason and he was re-admitted to hospital in September that year. I asked Dr P if Duncan could be seen by Dr Richardson. Dr P was very reluctant to allow this until Professor Basant Puri, a qualified Psychiatrist practising at Hammersmith Hospital, phoned Dr P and said that he would accompany Dr Richardson. Having examined Duncan, Dr Puri and Dr Richardson recommended that Duncan be put on high dose omega-3 supplements and amilsulpride instead of his usual neuroleptic drug, and that the dietary regime recommended by Dr Campbell-McBride be followed. They also requested that the tests into his physical health recommended by her be undertaken. We have never received the results of the tests and, some time later, we were told the results had been lost.

Dr P agreed to put Duncan on these supplements and amisulperide straight away. The dietary regime however, was not followed precisely. Despite this, Duncan made a recovery and was able to return to his flat a month later. During this time, I also spoke with Dr Abram Hoffer in Canada, who, together with Dr Humphrey Osmond, founded Orthomolecular Psychiatry, which uses nutritional supplements, such as vitamin B3, to cure symptoms of mental illness. He gave me a great deal of good advice.

In the meantime, I spent much time researching and found out that the human herpes virus 6 (HHV6) was implicated not only in chronic fatigue syndrome (CFS) and ME, but also in viral encephalitis, which in turn may trigger symptoms such as psychosis and paranoia. I contacted Dr Dharam Ablashi, Scientific Director of the HHV6 Foundation in the US and Kristen Loomis, Director, who told me that, given Duncan's childhood issues (severe roseola infection and learning difficulties), it was possible that he might have a chronic reactivation of HHV6 in his brain tissues and that this could represent the fundamental cause of his mental ill health. They explained that when HHV6 reactivates in transplant patients who are put on immune suppressants, they often develop central nervous system dysfunction and psychiatric problems.

The next time I saw Dr P, I told him about the HHV6 connection and asked if Duncan could be referred to a Virologist for tests. Later, I saw Dr P and he told me that he spoken with the Virologist who had dismissed the HHV6 virus connection to mental health as *'a load of American rubbish on the internet'* and was therefore unwilling to help. It was over a year later that I finally found a laboratory in the UK where they could test Duncan for HHV6 (his health had deteriorated dramatically as it had done every spring and autumn). The PCR test showed that he had a severe HHV6 infection. A private hospital used intravenous nutrients to boost Duncan's immune system to fight the HHV6 and we gave him an antiviral medicine based on information supplied by the HHV6 Foundation on protocols used in the US.

We have very recently been to see Dr Roberto Alvarez-La Fuente in Madrid, one of the world's leading experts on HHV6. Duncan has provided samples to determine his type of HHV6, which will determine what type of therapy he undertakes. In the UK, the doctors, having seen the private tests results showing that he had a leaky gut (leading to malabsorption of nutrients), yeast overgrowth and gluten intolerance, finally agreed that there would be benefit in giving Duncan a gastroscopy. This would determine if the last 10 months of intensive therapy had healed his gut.

I am happy to report that Duncan has now returned to full health after 10 months of intensive nutritional therapy, as well as extensive exposure to bright sunshine in

Spain to raise his vitamin D levels, on the advice of Mike Ash (vitamin D is an important antiviral). We have yet to see the results from Dr la Fuente, however, the results of the recent gastroscopy, show that Duncan's gut has healed. He still takes nutritional supplements including omega-3 oil for its antiviral effect and to repair the myelin damage caused by the HHV6 virus, as well as B vitamins, minerals, probiotics, L-Glutamine, the amino acid L-Lysine for it's anti-herpes properties, plus olive leaf extract, which is both antiviral and antifungal. These supplements enhance his immune system, fight infection and maintain the integrity of his gut. Finally, he remains on a very small dose (under the minimum recommended therapeutic dose) of amisulpride as advised by Professor Puri, until we can be sure from the outstanding tests that the factors underlying his previous condition have been cleared.

When Duncan was discharged from hospital last time, his diagnosis was changed from schizophrenia to *'non-organic psychosis of unknown origin'*. It is now clear that Duncan has suffered from an underlying viral infection (HHV6) since he was a toddler. It is likely that his use of cannabis triggered the mental health problems, as cannabis is a known immuno-suppressant. In addition, Duncan comes from an atopic family. Such families typically have conditions such as allergies to certain foods, asthma, eczema and often have higher requirements for certain nutrients. He also has a family history of diabetes. These facts were deliberately and consistently ignored and ridiculed by the psychiatric team responsible for Duncan's care. I was humiliated, ridiculed and ostracised for my determination to put forward reasons for and evidence of Duncan's illness.

There is no doubt in my mind that had I given up on my relentless quest to find the underlying causes of Duncan's condition and to explore all the combinations of factors that resulted in his illness, he would still be institutionalised. I watched my lively, creative, funny and highly popular young son disappear and didn't know if he would ever come back. I have been overwhelmed by the generosity of spirit and commitment to help by the many professionals that I have been in touch with throughout the world. The breath-taking arrogance, ignorance and dismissive attitude on the part of the 'professional' psychiatrists, and other doctors in charge of Duncan's care, caused me the deepest despair and sense of hopelessness. Most of all, they left me with an overwhelming sense of being disempowered and, therefore, helpless. As a result of this attitude Duncan was drugged into a stupor, unable to function with any sense of normality. We now know that this was entirely unnecessary.

Duncan has lost five of his most formative years and a great deal of confidence as a result. He has had to start over again. Thankfully, due to the severe tranquilising effect of the drugs administered to him, Duncan doesn't remember a lot of what happened. I recently asked Duncan what the past five years of illness had been like for him and he replied: *'Mum it's like I've woken up from a dream.'* For me, it's the beginning of the end of a five-year nightmare.

ACKNOWLEDGEMENTS

There is no doubt that Duncan would be in a long-term mental health institution were it not for the dedication, determination, knowledge, skills and, dare I say, love of the following people whose combined efforts brought Duncan back to full health:

■ Sally Bunday MBE, The Hyperactive Children's Support Group

■ Dr Yung Wei, Schizophrenia Association of Great Britain

■ Martina Watts

■ Dr Natasha Campbell-McBride

■ Dr Alex Richardson

■ Professor Basant Puri

■ Dr Abram Hoffer, Canada

■ Dr Dharam Ablashi, Scientific Director, HHV6 Foundation, US

■ Kristen Loomis, HHV6 Foundation, US

■ Brenda Queeley, Manager, Progress House

■ Lei Foster, Staff Nurse, Progress House

■ Dr P, Clinical Psychiatrist (who finally saw the light!)

■ Michael Ash

■ Frank McGowan.

Reference

Macpherson W (1999) *The Stephen Lawrence Inquiry/Report*. London: The Stationery Office.

Chapter 9
Orthomolecular medicine for schizophrenia
DR ABRAM HOFFER

Our use of vitamin B3 to treat schizophrenia was not serendipitous. It was based on our adrenochrome hypothesis, which pointed toward this vitamin and to antioxidants as a potential treatment. I became Director of Psychiatric Research, Department of Health in Saskatchewan, Canada in 1950. With my PhD in biochemistry and the MD I had an additional advantage – I knew no psychiatry. I had not been indoctrinated with the current belief that no cure would be found for this major disease. Half our mental hospital beds were filled with schizophrenics and an admission in 1950 was for life, with no time off for good behaviour (Hoffer, 2005a).

Fortunately, Dr H Osmond and his colleague Dr J Smythies in England had found that the experience induced by mescaline, one of the few then known hallucinogens, in many ways resembled the experience produced in normal people when they became schizophrenic. This idea was so repellent to the English establishment that Osmond fled to Saskatchewan and joined us as one of our superintendents. I looked at this hypothesis carefully, found it full of merit and then compared the chemical structure of all the hallucinogens: they were indoles or could become indoles in the body. The three of us then published our adrenochrome hypothesis, which suggested that schizophrenia might be caused by the excessive oxidation of adrenalin into adrenochrome. If this was indeed the case, it might be therapeutic to inhibit this reaction by using safe methods that could be taken for a lifetime in the same way that insulin can be used to treat diabetes mellitus (Hoffer *et al*, 1954; Hoffer and Osmond, 1967).

We decided to try niacin, one of the forms of vitamin B3, since it is a methyl acceptor and could deplete the body of methyl groups and decrease the conversion of noradrenalin to adrenalin, and there would therefore be less adrenalin to be oxidised to adrenochrome. Since the oxidation product of adrenaline is adrenochrome, we also used large doses of the natural antioxidant vitamin C to decrease the oxidation.

Our first clinical trials were encouraging and we proceeded to pilot studies. We had to determine how much to give and eventually settled on one gram after each of three meals as a starting dose. The first eight schizophrenic patients we treated at two of our hospitals recovered, or were much better. This led to our double-blind, prospective, randomised, controlled, therapeutic trials. With our first trial in 1953 we treated 30 schizophrenic patients. We were the first in psychiatry worldwide to do this type of study, which appears to be totally unknown to the psychiatric establishment. None of the patients were chronic patients in our mental hospitals. We suspected that early cases had a much better chance of responding. These were patients who were sick for the first time or who had been sick, got better and had relapsed again. We found that after a two-year follow-up, one-third of the placebo group was well and two-thirds of the vitamin group were well. Niacin and niacinamide were equally effective.

A second trial yielded the same results. The addition of one safe vitamin doubled the recovery rate for these schizophrenic patients. The only other treatment during the two trials was electro-convulsive therapy (ECT), which was also randomised but during the second, longer trial drugs had already been introduced and vitamins were not allowed. However, because of the use of drugs, it became increasingly difficult to find participants for trials as their psychiatrist wanted to put them all on drugs (Hoffer *et al*, 1957).

The treatment programme

There are three basic components of any treatment programme: shelter; nutritious food; treatment with respect and civility. Unfortunately, these are most often missing from modern psychiatry. The fourth component is orthomolecular psychiatry.

Shelter is obvious and need not be discussed. The quality of the food must be improved. The easiest way is to use the no-junk diet. I define 'junk' as any food to which sugar has been added. If these foods are excluded, this will also remove about 90% of other junk chemicals that are routinely added to our processed foods. This definition also includes refined cereals of any type.

In addition, many patients are mentally sick because they are allergic to one or more foods, usually staples. These can often be identified by their dietary history. The common foods are milk and any products derived from it, wheat, coffee, tea and more. If a food is suspected, it is eliminated. A young man, aged 22, complained that he had been depressed all his life. On the dairy elimination diet he was well in two weeks. He then ate ice cream. Two hours later, he was very depressed and one hour after that, he was agitated and psychotic. The police were called to restrain him. He fell asleep from 8.30pm to 11.30am and (off dairy) has been well since.

Nutrients most often used
Vitamin B3
(Hoffer and Foster, 2007)
There are two main forms of vitamin B3: nicotinic acid known medically as niacin and nicotinamide known as niacinamide. The term vitamin B3 refers to these two.

In some patients niacin will increase liver function test results. It is assumed, incorrectly, that elevated liver function test results always means underlying liver pathology. Usually, after a few days the test results become normal whether or not the niacin is still being taken. But to prevent confusing liver damage with increased activity, it is best to stop the niacin for five days and then do the tests (Hoffer, 2004).

The niacin flush or vasodilatation

Niacin usually causes a flush a few minutes after it is taken. A few people will flush with 25 mg, more with 50 mg and most with 100 mg. The flush begins in the forehead and works its way down the body, rarely affecting the toes. The higher the initial dose, the greater the initial flush, but if any dose causes a maximum flush, a larger dose taken later will not cause any greater flush. The capillaries are dilated and the blood flow through the organs is increased. Patients must be warned that this will happen. If they are not, they may be very surprised and even shocked. Patients can be started on lower doses until they have adjusted to the decreased intensity of the flush. Then the dose may be increased gradually.

Each time the niacin is taken, the flush is repeated, but to a much lesser degree. In most cases after a week or so it is almost all gone, and is a minor nuisance at worst. However, some people do not tolerate the flush and they will have to discontinue the niacin. For most conditions, the two forms (niacin and nicotinamide) are interchangeable. However, niacin normalises blood lipid levels and niacinamide does not.

The usual starting dose of niacin is 500–1,000 mg taken immediately after meals, three times daily. If one is worried about the intensity of the flush, one can start with 100 mg and increase it slowly. A few find this much more pleasant. Most patients will tolerate niacin if it is put to them in a positive way. Physicians who downplay its positive properties and emphasise its potential problems will find that most of their patients will not remain on it. Orthomolecular physicians find a very high compliance rate.

The dose of niacin seldom needs to go above two grams taken three times daily. It may be increased, but eventually the patient will develop nausea and later vomiting if the dose is too high and not decreased or stopped. The optimum dose range is very wide. The same doses are used with niacinamide, but the optimum dose range is narrower. More people develop nausea with niacinamide above six grams daily than with niacin. Children are more tolerant to these doses. The dose is not related to size, age or body weight. Some children will not complain of nausea but lose their appetite. Vitamin B3 must be given at least three times daily. It is water-soluble and very quickly excreted, making it very safe as the levels cannot build up, although this also means it has to be taken frequently and regularly.

Niacin and other medications

In common with all water-soluble nutrients, niacin is compatible with all foods and with medication. It reinforces the therapeutic effect of the antipsychotics, so that the dose of these powerful drugs can be reduced and fewer side effects will be experienced.

Vitamin B6: Pyridoxine

The dose ranges from 100–1,000 mg daily. The main indication is for those patients who excrete too much kryptopyrolle in their urine. Kryptopyrolle is excreted into the urine of many patients and a very few normal controls when they are under extreme pressure or increased oxidative stress. Both pyridoxine and zinc are used when this factor is present in excess (McGinnis *et al*, 2008). The usual dose of zinc is 50 mg of zinc citrate.

Ascorbic acid

Vitamin C (ascorbic acid) plays a major role in physical medicine. In mental illnesses it is not as relevant as the B vitamins, but due to its anti-stress properties, it is advantageous to use one to three grams daily for all patients. It is remarkably safe. The major side effect when large doses are used is loosening of the stools. This is not real diarrhoea as there is no pain or cramps. However, if these do occur, the dose should be decreased to below this level. The schizophrenia syndrome has occurred in scorbutic patients.

Essential fatty acids (EFAs)

The use of EFAs was proposed by Dr Donald Rudin over 15 years ago and amplified by Dr David Horrobin. A number of preparations are available. Usually patients need one to three grams of fish oil taken three times daily (Rudin and Felix, 1996; Horrobin, 1990).

Medication

This programme is entirely compatible with any medication. Most of the patients I see are already heavily medicated and have been on treatment for some time. The medication is maintained at the same level and the treatment programme is introduced. It takes about two months before the nutrient programme begins to show evidence of its effect. If the medication is reduced too early, the patient may relapse. But, after two months, if the patient is better or shows some evidence that the drugs are stronger, then they are very carefully and slowly decreased, consistent with good psychiatric practice.

The aim is to have the dose of medication so low that the patient is well with no side effects and, in many cases, if treatment is started early enough, the dose may be decreased to zero.

> Orthomolecular therapy does not mean that medication cannot be used. It is aimed at recovering the patients, no matter what has to be used, provided that the treatment is non-toxic and allows patients to recover.

Desiccated thyroid

In the past this natural thyroid hormone has been used with success in treating schizophrenia. It is not used today, because the standard is to depend entirely on laboratory tests, which can be misleading. Adrenochrome destroys thyroid tissue (Foster, 2003).

Results of treating schizophrenic patients

(Hoffer 1962; 1994; 1999; 2000; 2003; 2004; 2005a; 2005b; 2007a; Hoffer and Osmond, 1966; Hoffer *et al*, 1957)

Before discussing recovery it is necessary to define what this means. Recovery was not, and seldom is, expected in psychiatry when treating schizophrenia, and psychiatrists were content to record various degrees of improvement. The word cure does not appear in psychiatric dictionaries. Usually this meant that patients had fewer symptoms and were easier to deal with in hospital or at home. *To me, a patient is recovered when they are free of symptoms and signs, when they are getting on well with their family and in the community and when they are productive, employed and paying income tax.*

Recovery rates start at nearly zero per cent in the treatment given in the mental hospitals of the past between 1900 and 1950. None of the three basic conditions for recovery were used. The Quakers, with their moral treatment of the insane, claimed a 50% recovery rate. Dr John Connolly, using the same principles in England around 1840, found the same recovery rate, as did the early Dorothea Dix Hospitals in the US around the same time. If the same three factors are allowed to operate, it may be even higher, as a large number of patients suffering from mental illnesses remain undiagnosed and recover. We will never know how many of them were schizophrenic until we have an acceptable biochemical test for schizophrenia.

When the first three elements of recovery are not used, the recovery rate will be very low. When they are used at their optimum level, the rates will be at around 50%. This may explain the curious finding that patients who become schizophrenic in less-developed countries, like Bangladesh, have a better prognosis than similar patients who become ill in Canada or the US.

My conclusions of the results of treatment are based on double blind, controlled trials, on my own personal experience having treated over 5,000 patients since 1955 and on the results of numerous studies published by my colleagues over the past three decades, mostly in the *Journal of Orthomolecular Medicine* (JOM). (Medline refused to cover our journal; JOM is available online at: www.orthomolecular.org.)

If treated for up to two years, the recovery rate is about 90% for patients who have been sick for less than two years (or have been sick and recovered, then relapsed for less than two years).

The recovery rate for patients who have been sick longer than two years is not nearly as good. I found that about 50% of chronic patients, sick over seven years and treated for at least 10 years, recovered.

RECOVERY RATES

Mental hospital 1900 to 1950	0%
Modern psychiatry	<10%
Moral treatment	50%
Orthomolecular	75–90%

Source: Hoffer (2008) *Schizophrenia, Yesterday (1950) and Today: From despair to hope with orthomolecular psychiatry.* Victoria: Trafford.

ILLUSTRATIVE CASE HISTORY

The following case describes, in excellent detail, the outcome of treatment of one patient treated by his mother using the orthomolecular treatment. This one case, plus 18 additional personal accounts of patients who were treated successfully, illustrates how the orthomolecular approach is used and works (Hoffer, 2007b). A mother wrote the following about her son.

My 25-year-old son, John, was diagnosed with schizophrenia at the age of 15, suffering from both audio and visual hallucinations, in addition to extreme paranoia. He was also mutilating himself by burning and cutting, sometimes so seriously that emergency treatment was required. He believed that a dark 'higher power' was communicating with him, urging him to do harmful things to himself and others.

John was placed on the usual variety of medications, but each time he became stable, the drugs would have to be continually increased to maintain the same effect. John tried many different drugs over the years and these caused very troublesome side effects. The most disturbing were the facial tics and trembling that some of the antipsychotics caused. He also struggled with weight gain and fatigue.

Even on medication his life was miserable. John was never able to establish friendships, have a girlfriend, complete his education, or live on his own. The paranoia and delusions never completely went away, and John would often have panic attacks whenever he was in public with unfamiliar people.

When my father became ill and moved into our home, John helped to care for him. He gained the confidence to seek a career as a caregiver and took a short course to become a licensed certified nursing assistant (CNA). He was able to maintain employment for over three years in a nursing home with a low-stress environment. During that time, John was only hospitalised once, although he still had panic attacks and episodes of self-mutilation.

Around 18 months ago, John's schizophrenia became much worse and the medication was no longer able to control his symptoms. Since then, John has been placed in the local psychiatric hospital at least six times. He tried to kill himself by leaping in front of a moving truck, and also cut his wrist with a razor.

John was kept under a nearly constant watch by our entire family. John's psychiatrist felt that he needed to be placed in the state hospital for long-term treatment, but I resisted, urging the doctor to try different medications. In 2004, I came across the orthomolecular treatment for mental illness. At first, I didn't believe that something so simple could actually work, so didn't rush out to purchase the nutritional supplements.

Then John attempted suicide again, and I felt certain that if nothing changed, it was only a matter of time before John succeeded in taking his own life and maybe someone else's life as well. I started John on niacin. After the very first dose, the suicide attempts and self-mutilations stopped.

Before we began nutritional therapy, John was taking extremely high doses of medication daily and was still delusional, paranoid, suicidal and suffering panic attacks. He was taking daily:

- Effexor 600 mg
- Depakote 2,000 mg
- Zyprexa 10 mg
- Geodon 360 mg.

At first, the only supplement I tried was 500 mg of niacin. After the first two weeks he was up to 1,000 mg of niacin and his paranoia disappeared for the first time in over 10 years. Over the next few weeks we gradually increased the niacin to 3,000 mg per day and added other supplements, while gradually reducing his prescribed medications. John now takes daily:

- niacin 3,000 mg
- vitamin B6 400 mg
- omega-3 1,000 mg
- magnesium 100 mg
- zinc 15 mg
- vitamin C 1,000 mg.

He also takes a multivitamin and has drastically reduced his sugar and caffeine intake. His prescribed medications have been reduced to:

- Effexor 150 mg
- Depakote 500 mg
- Zyprexa 10 mg
- Geodon 240 mg.

We will continue to reduce these slowly over the next few weeks.

John is now free of all paranoia and delusions. In fact, he recently told me that he cannot believe the thoughts that were in his head before. For the first time in his life, he is able to feel comfortable in crowds and around strangers. I'm happy to report that John has been working as a CNA in a nursing home again for over a month and is talking about going back to school to become a licensed physical therapy assistant. He plans to move into his own apartment soon. John is now happy and hopeful about his future.

Update: 25 March 2005

I'd like to add an update to John's story. Over the past few weeks, he has continued to make great progress. He has continued reducing his prescription medications and has increased his niacin to 3.5 g daily. John is now completely off Depakote and, as a result, he has lost about 30 pounds. His facial ticks and trembling have almost completely disappeared.

John has not had even one episode of suicidal feelings, self-mutilation or panic attacks. He is usually in a very positive state of mind and is very excited about his future. He is becoming much more independent and learning to handle life's challenges without my assistance.

One big achievement is that John finally remembers to take his supplements and medications on his own. Our whole family had taken on the responsibility of making certain that John took his medication twice daily because he would simply forget to take it. Now, I don't even think about reminding John because he always remembers it himself. Basically, John has his life back now. He was able to accomplish this by taking supplements along with his medication. We hope that he will eventually be off the prescription drugs entirely, but we are taking small steps towards that direction.

Editor's comment

Orthomolecular psychiatry is a highly specialised area and is based on an individual's biochemical requirements. The nutrient dosages suggested here are beyond usual recommended daily allowances. Expert medical advice should be sought before taking any high dose vitamin and mineral supplements, particularly if they are taken for an extended period of time.

References

Foster HD (2003) *What Really Causes Schizophenia*. Victoria BC: Trafford Press. Available at: www.hdfoster.com

Hoffer A (1962) *Niacin Therapy in Psychiatry*. Springfield: CC Thomas.

Hoffer A (1994) Chronic schizophrenic patients treated ten years or more. *Journal of Orthomolecular Medicine* **9** (1) 7–37.

Hoffer A (1999) *Orthomolecular Treatment for Schizophrenia*. New Canaan: Keats Publishing.

Hoffer A (2000) *Vitamin B-3 and Schizophrenia: Discovery, recovery, controversy*. Kingston: Quarry Press.

Hoffer A (2003) Negative and positive side effects of vitamin B-3. *Journal of Orthomolecular Medicine* **18** 146–160.

Hoffer A (2004) *Healing Schizophrenia*. Toronto: CCNM Press.

Hoffer A (2005a) *Adventures in Psychiatry*. Toronto: Kos Press.

Hoffer A (2005b) *Healing Children's Attention and Behavior Disorders*. Toronto: CCNM Press.

Hoffer A (2007a) *Mental Health Regained*. Toronto: International Schizophrenia Foundation.

Hoffer A (2007b) *Treatment Manual*. Toronto: International Schizophrenia Foundation.

Hoffer A and Foster HD (2007) *Feel Better, Live Longer With Vitamin B-3*. Toronto: CCNM Press.

Hoffer A and Osmond H (1966) *How To Live With Schizophrenia*. New York: University Books.

Hoffer A and Osmond H (1967) *The Hallucinogens*. New York: Academic Press.

Hoffer A, Osmond H and Smythies J (1954) Schizophrenia: A new approach II. Results of a year's research. *Journal of Mental Science* **100** (418) 29–45.

Hoffer A, Osmond H, Callbeck MJ and Kahan I (1957) Treatment of schizophrenia with nicotinic acid and nicotinamide. *Journal of Clinical and Experimental Psychopathology and Quarterly Review of Psychiatry and Neurology* **18** (2) 131–158.

Horrobin DF (1990) *Omega-6 Essential Fatty Acids: Pathophysiology and roles in clinical medicine*. New York: Wiley-Liss.

McGinnis WR, Audhya T, Walsh WJ, Jackson JA, McLaren-Howard J, Lewis A, Lauda P, Bibus DM, Jurnak F, Lietha R and Hoffer A (2008) Discerning the mauve factor alternative medicine in health and medicine. *Alternative Therapies in Health and Medicine* **14** (3).

Rudin D and Felix C (1996) *Omega-3 Oils: A practical guide*. New York: Avery.

Chapter 10
The effect of food intolerance and allergy on mood and behaviour

ANTONY J HAYNES

The subject of food intolerance and its impact on mental health is both controversial and complex. This chapter can, therefore, only summarise the fundamental issues involved.

Historical perspective

There is no mention at all in standard textbooks on neurology and psychiatry of any connection with mental illness and adverse reactions to food or, indeed, chemicals or inhalants.

However, a group of psychiatrists, termed orthomolecular-ecologic psychiatrists, believe that the fundamental cause of a range of mental and emotional illnesses is the food eaten by the patient, the chemicals they are exposed to, inhaled allergies, addictions and other non-immunologic maladaptive reactions. They believe that patients with mental illness should be assessed for *'brain allergies'* (Philpott and Kalita, 2000).

Among the ranks of orthomolecular-ecologic psychiatrists are Drs Klotz, Mandell, Randolph, Shurley, Rowe, Duke, Hoffer, Kennedy, Davidson, Alvarez, Clark and Rinkel. The work of PhD chemists such as Drs Khaleeluddin and Rubin has also proven invaluable.

In 1970 Dr Frederic Speer wrote a book entitled *Allergy of the Nervous System*, and described how emotional and neurological symptoms (from allergy and neurology sources) have been observed and recorded since the 1920s. Even earlier, in 1916, Dr Hoobler reported that infants can be intolerant to certain proteins (Hoobler, 1916). Indeed, the association of symptoms with certain foods goes much further back than the 20th century, with Heroditus in 460 BC stating that *'one man's food is another's poison'*.

Despite the evidence, the focus on food's link with mental health appears to have been largely overlooked. The eminent US ecologist Dr Theron Randolph believes that 60–70% of symptoms diagnosed as psychosomatic are, in fact, reactions to foods, chemicals and inhalants.

Dr William Philpott emphasises that it is the underlying organic cause of mental illness that is important. He writes:

'We should be diagnosing paranoia caused by a wheat allergy, dissociation as a manifestation of mold or hydrocarbon allergy, and so forth, according to people's specific reactions to individual foods, chemicals and inhalants.'
(Philpott and Kalita, 2000)

Physicians who are aware of food intolerance, and experienced in diagnosing it, estimate that 20–30% of psychosomatic symptoms may be traced to adverse reactions to food. However, this is not to say that all patients in mental hospitals are there because of undiagnosed food sensitivity. Nonetheless, it would appear logical to rule out the influence of food intolerances in someone with mood or behaviour conditions.

Research evidence

There is much good evidence, including double-blind studies, of the association of food allergy and intolerance and its negative effect on the nervous system, mood and behaviour (Duke, 1923; MacKarness, 1979; Randolph, 1962; Davison, 1949; Rinkel, 1944; Speer, 1954; Roth, 1978; Pfeiffer, 1987; Schauss, 1981; Randolph, 1945; Kittler and Baldwin, 1970; Swanson, 1978; Rinkel *et al*, 1951; Moyer, 1975; King and Mandell, 1978; Miller, 1977; Feingold, 1975; Egger *et al*, 1985; O'Shea and Porter, 1981; Boris and Mande, 1994).

There is evidence showing a link between a subgroup of people suffering with anxiety and depression and irritable bowel syndrome (IBS) and food allergy (Addolorato *et al*, 1998; Marshall, 1993; Djuric *et al*, 1995). Depression has also been linked with low back pain (Hurwitz and Morgenstern, 1999). The expression to convey this state of inflammation-induced depression, in animals and humans, has been called *'cytokine-induced sickness'* (Dunn *et al*, 2005; Dantzer, 2001).

Some researchers claim that attention deficit hyperactivity disorder (ADHD) is caused by inadequate production of the neurotransmitter dopamine, which may be due to a genetic predisposition exacerbated by certain foods. The researchers identify that:

'An understanding of the interactive responses involved in the neuroendocrine-immunological network is essential for a comprehension of the pathophysiology of ADHD, CFS (chronic fatigue syndrome), and FM (fibromyalgia) and the role of allergies appears to be an important triggering event in each of the disorders.'
(Bellanti et al, 2005)

What is the difference between food allergy and intolerance?

The incidence of food allergies is increasing. In the US allergy is ranked as the sixth leading cause of chronic disease today, with over 50 million sufferers from one type or another (American Academy of Allergy, Asthma and Immunology (AAAAI),

1996–2001). In the UK, it is estimated that 18 million people have at least one allergy (Surrey Allergy Clinic, online) and nearly 28 million people have an intolerance (Breath Spa For Kids, 2007).

Food allergy is probably best defined as an abnormal immunological reaction to food. This means that if an individual is exposed to a food they are allergic to, an immune response occurs that can be measured in the blood. The response is swift, usually within 30 minutes, clearly defined and reproducible. It classically involves the production of special antibodies to foods called IgE. Swollen lips or eyelids are typical manifestations, along with digestive complaints occurring rapidly after consumption. Allergy to peanuts is probably the best known, with even a trace of peanut eliciting an immediate and potentially life-threatening response (anaphylaxis). The most common foods causing anaphylactic shock are nuts, milk, some kinds of fruit, fish and, less commonly, spices.

Latex, bee or wasp stings and a number of drugs, especially penicillins, painkillers, anaesthetic drugs, dyes and intravenous infusion liquids can produce similar reactions.

Oral allergy syndrome (OAS) is another immunological (rarely anaphylactic) condition that manifests in patients with an allergy to pollen. The immune system mistakes food proteins for pollen proteins, triggering an allergic reaction. Symptoms include itching and tingling with or without oedema of the lips, mouth and tongue after eating fresh fruits and vegetables (Tishida *et al*, 2000). Certain fruits and vegetables are associated with reactivity to certain pollens, such as apple, carrot, pear, cherry with birch pollen, and tomato, melon, watermelon with grass pollen (Ortolani *et al*, 1988). Cooking or canning of food tends to reduce the reactivity of the antigen.

ANTIBODIES AND ANTIGENS

> Antibodies are types of protein produced by white blood cells. They react with, protect against and help destroy foreign substances called antigens. An antigen is a protein that may be a micro-organism (bacteria, virus, fungus), or a toxin given off by an invading micro-organism, chemical or fragment of food, usually a protein. The body makes five distinct classes of antibodies in response to specific antigens: IgA; IgD; IgE; IgG; IgM. The 'Ig' stands for immunoglobulin (an alternative name for antibody). IgE is involved in allergic reactions, whereas IgG responds to any foreign body invasion and is the most abundant.

Food intolerance

Food intolerance is also an adverse reaction to a specific food or food ingredient. However, food intolerance is not necessarily associated with clearly defined immune reactions in the same way as food allergy, and may involve a number of different reactions including mood and behaviour. It has been estimated that as many as 80% of food intolerances involve IgG reactions.

IgE, IgG and other types of antibodies are found in the gut wall and release inflammatory messengers including histamine. This has the effect of altering the permeability of the gut, making it more 'leaky'. As a consequence, food can be absorbed when it has only been partly digested and large, unrecognised food molecules, called peptides, may enter the bloodstream. These then trigger a number of immune responses, usually some time after the food was eaten, causing many of the unpleasant symptoms seen in food intolerance. One of the key differences between allergy and intolerance to food is the speed of response – allergy is immediate, whereas intolerance can be delayed for as long as 72 hours.

Localised secretory immunoglobulin A (SIgA) is responsible for protecting mucosal surfaces and provides the first immune response to antigens that are consumed. People with lowered levels of SIgA are more likely to suffer from increased intestinal permeability and an increased uptake of food antigens (Ahmed and Fuchs, 1997).

Food intolerance not only affects the body, but also mental health, mood and behaviour. Symptoms can occur on a regular basis, as often as every day, but may not be understood to be related to food. The following symptoms have all been associated with food intolerance and allergy (Haynes, 2005).

SYMPTOMS ASSOCIATED WITH FOOD INTOLERANCE

- Addictions
- Aggressive outbursts
- Anxiety
- ADD/ADHD
- Anxiety
- Behavioural problems
- Blankness or momentary difficulty in finding the right word(s)
- Blurred vision
- Brain fog
- Changes in handwriting
- Clumsiness
- Confusion
- Constant hunger
- Dark circles under eyes
- Depression
- Dilated blood vessels in cheeks and nose
- Dizziness
- Dyslexia
- Epileptic seizures
- Foggy head

- Food cravings
- Headaches
- Hyperactivity (especially in children)
- Inability to think clearly
- Insomnia
- Irritability
- Lack of motivation/get up and go
- Migraines
- Mood swings
- Palpitations
- Panic attacks
- Phobias
- Poor concentration
- Racing pulse
- Restless legs syndrome
- Schizophrenia
- Slurred speech
- Spacey
- Tenseness
- Tinnitus (ringing in the ears)
- Uncharacteristic inability to make decisions

Food intolerance is largely ignored by the NHS. Even in the field of allergy, there are relatively few specialists in the NHS, given its prevalence. However, even on one NHS website (NHS allergy site quiz, online), there is reference to at least a couple of 'brain' effects caused by food intolerance. The quiz suggests that if the answer to any of these questions is 'yes', then there may be a food intolerance involved. Only six symptoms are listed, compared to the 40 opposite, but note that fatigue, tiredness and craving are included.

NHS ALLERGY SITE QUIZ

Do you regularly experience any of these symptoms?
- Bloating and pain in your tummy
- Diarrhoea and/or constipation
- Wind or grumbling tummy
- Tiredness or lack of energy
- Headache or migraine
- Craving for common foods, such as wheat (bread, pasta) or dairy foods

Who is affected by food intolerance?

It is estimated that 45% of the population has at least one food intolerance (Breath Spa For Kids, 2007), which is considerably greater than those suffering an IgE allergy in their lifetime (Asthma and Allergy Information and Research (AAIR), online). However, because the reaction within the body is not confined to a single immunological antibody, it is not straightforward to determine or test the presence of food intolerance in the population. Given this lack of clarity, it is simply not known to what extent these produce physical symptoms or changes in mood and behaviour.

As a result of consumer concerns, the UK free-from food market, including dairy-, gluten- and wheat-free products, has already enjoyed sales growth of over 300% since 2000 and is set to double, according to market analyst Mintel (Health24, online).

Mood and behaviour: the most common offenders

The most common offending foods to trigger mood and behaviour problems are: wheat and other gluten grains (rye, barley, oats), corn, cows' milk, certain food additives and colouring, and tobacco (Philpott and Kalita, 2000).

MOST COMMON OFFENDERS

- Wheat
- Cows' milk
- Other gluten grains (rye, barley and possibly oats)
- Corn
- Food additives
- Artificial colourings
- Tobacco

A word about gluten

A prime candidate thought to trigger or cause mental and emotional symptoms is gluten. Symptoms include anxiety, depression, obsessions, phobias, compulsive behaviours and even hallucinations and delusions (Philpott and Kalita, 2000).

There has been some indication that those suffering from the autoimmune condition coeliac disease, which requires the complete avoidance of gluten in the diet, are significantly more likely to also suffer from schizophrenia. However, this remains controversial, with some studies showing no increased incidence in the coeliac population compared to a normal (ie. non-coeliac) population (Stevens *et al*, 1977; West *et al*, 2006). More recently, researchers have identified an increased incidence of non-affective psychosis in those suffering from coeliac disease (Ludvigsson *et al*, 2007). Careful case history and assessment is required in each case.

Other known offenders

There are countless foods and other substances that may cause adverse reactions in people and this is why it is so important to be assessed by a practitioner who is skilled in taking case histories and in the assessment of food allergy and intolerance. Almost any commonly consumed food could be a culprit; the following chemicals in particular need to be considered: amines; salicylates; artificial colours; natural colour annatto (E160b); sorbates; benzoates; sulphites; propionates; nitrates; synthetic antioxidants; MSG and MSG-free flavour enhancers. To make matters even more complicated, it may not be the food itself that elicits a reaction, but pesticides or other chemicals sprayed onto it.

Caffeine

Excess caffeine can produce a variety of symptoms that are not as likely to be food intolerance related, but due to the direct stimulatory effect on the central nervous system. These include anxiety, mood swings, excessive perspiration, irregular heartbeat, palpitations, tremors and insomnia.

Addiction

It is estimated that half of people with food intolerances have cravings for those same foods they react to. It is thought that the mechanism behind the addictive aspect of food intolerance involves endorphins, which are our natural opioids. When the effect wears off, the person is more likely to crave the food that elicited this effect, hence the addictive nature of foods to which one has an intolerance.

How do you know if you have a food intolerance?

If you suspect that you or a patient has food intolerances that may be affecting mood and behaviour, what is the best method of determining whether this is true?

There are a number of different ways, and each may be equally valid to the individual:

- observation
- laboratory testing
- elimination diet
- pulse testing.

Observation

Even simple observation is scientific. The observation that a certain food or foods precipitates symptoms, in a predictable fashion, may be enough to confirm that it is 'real'. The suspect foods then need to be avoided for a period of time. Given the nature of the delayed reaction of food intolerances, as compared to immediate allergies, it is not always possible to determine culprit foods. The foods or substances on the main culprit list are wheat and other gluten grains, dairy, corn, food additives and colourings, and tobacco (ie. smokers). In addition, many people react to sugar and yeast, which may be due to gut dysbiosis. A review of the diet can readily identify whether these items are consumed in large amounts.

Laboratory evidence

The most reliable way of confirming culprit foods is by challenge under medical supervision (Sampson, 1999). The testing of food intolerances is a highly controversial area, with questions about its reproducibility and accuracy. One also has to consider the huge variety of different mechanisms that could potentially trigger unusual reactions. One of the most accurate and reproducible methods of food intolerance testing is via a method called ELISA (Enzyme Linked ImmunoSorbent Assay). This is particularly useful for detecting additives that may be missed by other techniques, and of particular importance in affecting mood and behaviour (IWDL Genova Diagnostics, online; Cambridge Nutritional Sciences, online).

About 90% of food intolerances are non-IgE mediated, and the majority of these are estimated to be mediated by an IgG reaction (Direct Laboratory Services, online). Simply because there is no IgE allergy does not mean that there is not an IgG or, indeed, a non-IgG reaction.

For some people, the testing of over 100 foods is the best frontline method of determining which foods need to be avoided. It is rare for someone to have just one food intolerance, although there may be one or two major foods that provoke symptoms.

Elimination or diversified rotation diet

This approach could form the mainstay of action to help overcome the negative effects on mood and behaviour caused by foods. It can be used once food intolerances have been diagnosed, or as a method of determining which foods are causing symptoms. There are a variety of elimination diets under different names. The approach aims to reduce the variety of foods consumed to a minimum, while avoiding all the usual suspects, and then re-introduces foods one at a time, with a delay between one food and another in order to determine if symptoms are triggered.

Over the years, there have been revisions of the diversified rotation diet and a standard of excellence has been developed by Dr Theron Randolph who describes the three main points of the diet.

1. Any one food, whether initially symptom-reactive or not, should be eaten only once in four days.

2. Foods are established in families, with only one member of any family eaten during any one day.

3. One day must intervene between the use of any two members of a food family.

The doctors and allergists involved in implementing these diets, which require no small amount of hard work, emphasise that a symptom-producing food does not have to be avoided forever, but can be returned to the diet after the body has had time to recover completely from the initial allergic reaction. The typical timeframe for the length of avoidance is three months for a minor reaction, and longer for foods that elicit stronger reactions.

The specific detail and intricate nature of planning an elimination and rotation diet means that anyone intending to follow this approach needs to seek the advice of a healthcare professional trained in this area.

Pulse testing

Over 50 years ago, Dr Arthur Coca devised a method of pulse testing described in his book *The Pulse Test: Easy allergy detection* (Coca, 1956). It is a method to be tried and tested, and should be used more often. This is a simple, yet extremely effective way to identify foods to which a patient may be sensitive. Simply put, stress will cause the pulse to increase. Foods to which you are intolerant cause physiological stress and will reveal themselves by speeding up your pulse. Through this test, Dr Coca was able to eliminate a myriad of symptoms and conditions simply by identifying and eliminating from the diet, foods to which the patient was intolerant.

Action steps

Seek the help of a nutrition practitioner who is experienced in both the identification of food intolerances and allergy and in taking a detailed case history. There are then seven steps to follow.

1. **Identify food allergies/intolerances**, either with laboratory testing, observation or pulse testing. Discuss with the practitioner the most appropriate one for you.

2. **Exclude foods that are causing symptoms** and reintroduce later. It is extremely important to ensure that whole major food groups are not avoided and to follow a common-sense healthy eating approach (ie. no refined sugar, cigarettes, recreational drugs, alcohol) even if these are not evidently things to which there exists an intolerance or allergy. Again, please consult an experienced health professional.

3. **Support digestion** with the tools of nutritional therapy.

   - Chew food thoroughly because it starts off the digestive process and naturally increases the production of epithelial growth factor, which helps to support the renewal of the gut lining.

   - Assess the status of hydrochloric acid (HCl) in the stomach. HCl is vital in the process of digestion and commences the breakdown of proteins. When this does not occur, there is increased risk of food intolerance. Pancreatic enzymes complete the job of protein digestion. Nutritional therapists can advise on the provision, for a period of time, of HCl and digestive enzymes for those individuals who require them.

   - If there is an imbalance in the bacteria or yeast within the gut, this also needs addressing as it contributes to an increased risk of inflammation, maldigestion and altered intestinal permeability. Targeted probiotic therapy can be of utmost importance.

   - The integrity of the gut lining can become compromised. Contributing factors include maldigestion, imbalanced gut flora, drugs (antibiotics, NSAIDs) and stress. The so-called 'leaky gut' is known to increase the incidence of food intolerance. Nutritional therapists can advise on diet and specific nutrients to heal the gut lining.

4. **Support the immune system**, as stress, certain drugs and other factors can adversely affect levels of our immune defences, such as the protective secretory immunoglobulin A (SIgA) – this increases the risk of food intolerance. SIgA levels can be tested for, and nutritional therapy can help to restore optimal levels.

5. **Identify imbalances** in other aspects of health. Having a bad back is a good example. Aim to correct this because it may affect and increase the risk of food intolerance (for example if patients are taking NSAIDs), and almost certainly increases the prevalence of inflammatory cytokines.

6. **Support liver detoxification**, as by supporting liver detoxification pathways, there is less risk of inflammatory molecules entering the bloodstream and consequently affecting the brain. An experienced practitioner will be in a position to assess which type of liver support is required.

7. **Embrace healthy living habits**, including ensuring adequate sleep, living in a tidy environment without too much noise or artificial lighting, gentle exercise outdoors every day where possible, spending time with friends, and doing things that make you laugh.

References

Addolorato G, Marsigli L, Capristo E, Caputo F, Dall'Aglio C and Baudanza P (1998) Anxiety and depression: a common feature of health care seeking patients with irritable bowel syndrome and food allergy. *Hepatogastroenterology* **45** (23) 1559–1564.

Ahmed T and Fuchs GJ (1997) Gastrointestinal allergy to food: a review. *Journal of Diarrhoeal Diseases Research* **15** (4) 211–223.

American Academy of Allergy, Asthma and Immunology (AAAAI) (1996–2001) *The Allergy Report: Science based findings on the diagnosis and treatment of allergic disorders.* Milwaukee: American Academy of Allergy, Asthma and Immunology.

Asthma and Allergy Information and Research (AAIR) [online] available at: http://www.users.globalnet.co.uk/~aair/anaphylaxis.htm#SEC1 [accessed 20/1/08].

Bellanti JA, Sabra A, Castro HJ, Chavez JR,J Malka-Rais J and de Inocencio JM (2005) Are attention deficit hyperactivity disorder and chronic fatigue syndrome allergy related? What is fibromyalgia? *Allergy and Asthma Proceedings* **26** (1) 19–28.

Boris M and Mande FS (1994) Food and additives are common causes of the attention deficit hyperactive disorder in children. *Annals of Allergy* **72** 462–468.

Breath Spa For Kids (2007) *Food Allergy and Intolerance Week in the UK* [online] available at: http://breathspakids.blogspot.com/2007/01/food-allergy-and-intolerance-week-in.html [accessed 20/1/08].

Cambridge Nutritional Sciences, Cambridgeshire. Web: www.cambridge-nutritional.com/Scripts/whatis.asp; Email: Labtests@cambridge-nutritional.com; Tel: 01353 863279; Fax: 01353 863330.

Coca AF (1956) *The Pulse Test: Easy allergy detection.* New York: Arco Publishing.

Dantzer R (2001) Part IV: cytokines, chronic fatigue states, and sickness behavior: cytokine-induced sickness behavior: mechanisms and implications. *Annals of the New York Academy of Sciences* **933** 222–234.

Davison HM (1949) Cerebral allergy. *Southern Medical Journal* **42** (8) 712.

Direct Laboratory Services. Web: www.directlabs.com/ImmunoLabs.php [accessed: 16/02/08].

Djuric VJ, Overstreet DH, Bienenstock J and Perdue MH (1995) Immediate hypersensitivity in the Flinders rat: further evidence for a possible link between susceptibility to allergies and depression. *Brain, Behavior, and Immunity* **9** (3) 196–206.

Duke WW (1923) Meniere's syndrome caused by allergies. *Journal of the American Medical Association* **81** 2179–2181.

Dunn AJ, Swiergiel AH and de Beaurepaire R (2005) Cytokines as mediators of depression: what can we learn from animal studies? *Neuroscientists and Behavioral Reviews* **29** (4–5) 891–909.

Egger J, Carter C, Graham P, Gumley D and Soothill J (1985) Controlled trial of oligoantigenic treatment in the hyperkinetic syndrome. *The Lancet* **325** 540–345.

Feingold N (1975) *Why Your Child is Hyperactive.* New York: Random House.

Haynes A (2005) *The Food Intolerance Bible.* London: Harper Collins.

Health24 [online] *Allergy vs Intolerance* available at: www.health24.com/dietnfood/Allergy_intolerance/15-3110-3112-3125,37275.asp [accessed 20/1/08].

Hoobler BR (1916) Some early symptoms suggesting protein sensitization in infancy. *American Journal of Diseases of Children* **12** 129.

Hurwitz EL and Morgenstern H (1999) Cross-sectional associations of asthma, hay fever, and other allergies with major depression and low-back pain among adults aged 20–39 years in the United States. *American Journal of Epidemiology* **150** (10) 1107–1116.

IWDL Genova Diagnostics, Surrey. Web: www.iwdl.net/tests.htm; Email: info@iwdl.net or kitorders@iwdl.net; Tel: 020 8336 7750; Fax: 020 8336 7751.

King DS and Mandell M (1978) *A Double-blind Study of Allergic Cerebral-viscero-somatic Malfunctions Evoked by Provocative Sublingual Challenges with Allergic Extracts: Statistical confirmation of the induction of psychological (mental) and somatic symptoms by provocative testing.* Proceedings of the 12th Advanced Seminar in Clinical Ecology, Key Biscayne, October 1978. See also: King DS (1979) *Effects of Sublingual Testing: A double-blind study.* Proceedings of the 13th Advanced Seminar in Clinical Ecology, San Diego, October 1979.

Kittler FJ and Baldwin DG (1970) The role of allergic factors in the child with minimal brain dysfunction. *Annals of Allergy* **23** 203–206.

Ludvigsson JF, Osby U, Ekbom A and Montgomery SM (2007) Coeliac disease and risk of schizophrenia and other psychosis: a general population cohort study. *Scandinavian Journal of Gastroenterology* **42** (2) 179–185.

MacKarness R (1979) *Eating Dangerously: The hazards of hidden allergies.* New York: Harcourt Brace Jovanovich.

Marshall PS (1993) Allergy and depression: a neurochemical threshold model of the relation between the illnesses. *Psychological Bulletin* **113** (1) 23–43.

Miller JB (1977) A double-blind study of food extract injection therapy: a preliminary report. *Annals of Allergy* **38** 185–191.

Moyer KE (1975) The physiology of violence: allergy and aggression. *Psychology Today* July 76–79.

NHS allergy site quiz available online at: http://www.nhs.uk/magazines/allergies/Pages/QuizFoodIntolerance.aspx [accessed 20/01/08].

Ortolani C, Ispano M, Pastorello E, Bigi A and Ansaloni R (1988) The oral allergy syndrome. *Annals of Allergy* **61** (6 part 2) 47–52.

O'Shea J and Porter S (1981) Double-blind study of children with hyperkinetic syndrome treated with multi-allergen extract sublingually. *Journal of Learning Disabilities* **14** (4) 189–191.

Pfeiffer CC (1987) *Nutrition and Mental Illness.* Rochester: Healing Arts Press.

Philpott WH and Kalita DK (2000) *Brain Allergies* (2nd edition). New Canaan: Keats Publishing.

Randolph TG (1945) Fatigue and weakness of allergic origin (allergic toxemia) to be differentiated from nervous fatigue and neurasthenia. *Annals of Allergy* **3** 418–430.

Randolph TG (1962) *Human Ecology and Susceptibility to the Chemical Environment.* Springfield: Charles C Thomas.

Rinkel HJ (1944) Food allergy: the role of food allergy in internal medicine. *Annals of Allergy* **2** 115–124.

Rinkel HJ, Randolph TG and Zeller M (1951) *Food Allergy.* Springfield: Charles C Thomas.

Roth J (1978) *The Food/Depression Connection: Dietary control of allergy-based mood swings.* Chicago: Contemporary Books.

Sampson HA (1999) Food allergy, part two: diagnosis and management. *Journal of Allergy and Clinical Immunology* **103** (6) 981–989.

Schauss A (1981) *Diet, Crime and Delinquency.* Berkeley: Parker House.

Speer F (1954) Allergic tension-fatigue in children. *Annals of Allergy* **12** 168–171.

Speer G (1970) *Allergy of the Nervous System.* Springfield: Charles C Thomas.

Stevens FM, Lloyd RS, Geraghty SM, Reynolds MT, Sarsfield MJ, Mcnicholl B, Fottrell PF, Wright R and Mccarthy CF (1977) Schizophrenia and coeliac disease – the nature of the relationship. *Psychological Medicine* **7** (2) 259–263.

Surrey Allergy Clinic [online] available at: www.allergy-clinic.co.uk/index.html [accessed 10/2/08].

Swanson J (1978) *Behavioural Responses to Artificial Colour.* Presented at the 2nd International Food Allergy Symposium, American College of Allergists, Mexico City, Mexico.

Tishida, K Murai, T Yasuda, T Satou, T Sejima and Kitamura K (2000) Oral allergy syndrome in patients with Japanese cedar pollinosis. *Nippon Jibiinkoka Gakkai Kaiho* **103** (3) 199–205.

West J, Logan RF, Hubbard RB and Card TR (2006) Risk of schizophrenia in people with coeliac disease, ulcerative colitis and Crohn's disease: a general population-based study. *Alimentary Pharmacology and Therapeutics* **23** (1) 71–74.

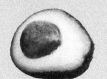

Chapter 11
Blood sugar blues

KATE NEIL

Regulation of blood glucose is arguably the most important nutritional intervention in clinical practice today. Increasingly, the scientific data supports a causal role for insulin sensitivity problems in a wide spectrum of modern degenerative diseases including: obesity, cardiovascular disease, type 2 diabetes, stroke, certain types of cancer and polycystic ovary syndrome (PCOS) (Bland and Jones, 2006).

Depression secondary to chronic illness is common and, although this may be partly explained by social circumstances, more attention on supporting blood glucose control would be likely to improve the mental well-being of sufferers.

Many people are familiar with the yo-yo effects of poor blood glucose regulation and choose foods and stimulants that help keep the unwanted symptoms of sugar dips at bay. We quickly learn that a strong coffee and a cigarette can help to keep us going, tea and biscuits mid-morning will give us a lift and the chocolate bar mid-afternoon will relieve us of the 'sugar blues'.

Dietary macro- and micronutrients are important regulators of glucose balance and a range of nutritional supplements and botanicals have also been shown to be helpful. In addition, exercise and stress management are integral lifestyle components of a successful nutritional therapy programme to support blood glucose balance.

Compliance, both short and long term, to diet and lifestyle change is frequently problematic and many studies and surveys confirm this finding. Education and advice is often not enough to bring about sustainable change. Even when life itself is imminently threatened, implementing and sustaining change can be challenging.

Since the long-term health implication of dysregulated blood glucose is far-reaching – affecting mental health as well as many degenerative diseases – the skills required of all health professionals go beyond their basic training. Acquiring coaching skills is fundamental to facilitating change in beliefs and attitudes that can block an individual's road to progress and improved health.

There is no better time to start the process of the expression of health than working with couples who plan to have a baby. A dramatic reduction in many chronic health problems would be likely to occur if more parents became aware of the importance of modifying their diets and lifestyles prior to conception and maintained positive changes long term (Barker, 1994).

In the meantime, health practitioners have a hard task ahead of them – to not only support their patients in establishing healthy diet and lifestyle practices, but will also often need professional support to apply the same principles in their own lives.

The body is designed to tightly control the level of glucose in the bloodstream. Normally the pancreas secretes the right amount of insulin to adequately clear glucose from the bloodstream. In the average adult, five to six grams of glucose (the equivalent of about a small commercial sugar packet added to tea) circulates in about five litres of blood (for a Wikipedia definition, see http://en.wikipedia.org/wiki/Blood_sugar). This is enough to supply the energy required for all the processes in the body that depend on glucose. Glucose in excess of what the body immediately requires is stored in cells for later use.

The 'Western diet' and lifestyle

The 'Western diet' is strongly associated with dysregulated blood sugar. In terms of the macronutrients, the research literature increasingly demonstrates that diets 'high' in protein and low in simple carbohydrates, providing a balance of beneficial fats, would best support glucose control (Linkner, 2007).

Many changes have occurred as a result of the industrial revolution, including the increased consumption of refined grain and refined sugar. Large nutrient losses occur as a result of refining foods including: B vitamins, chromium, magnesium and zinc. All of these nutrients have a role to play in managing blood sugar levels. Fibre has a significant role in blood sugar control and is lost during the refining process.

The way meals are balanced has shifted over the last 50 or more years. Breakfasts are structured more around cereals with added sugar and skimmed or lower fat milk, bread, preserves, fruit and fruit juices or smoothies; lunch around sandwiches, paninis or baguettes devoid of vegetables, containing little protein and filled with mayo or other sauce and butter or margarine; pasta, white rice or potato often forms a substantial part of an evening meal; cakes, biscuits and confectionery are common snacks or eaten instead of meals; fizzy drinks, cordials and alcohol are regularly consumed. The coffee-bar culture is growing in Britain. As well as the stimulating effects of caffeine, many special coffees are very sweet and loaded in unnecessary calories.

Glycaemic index and glycaemic load

The above is vastly different to the meat-and-two-veg or go-to-work-on-an-egg concepts that prevailed pre and post war or a hearty bowl of porridge oats. In 1981 David Jenkins developed the 'glycaemic index (GI)' to measure the rise of blood glucose after eating a particular food (Jenkins *et al*, 1981). More recently, the concept of 'glycaemic load (GL)' has emerged (Brand-Miller *et al*, 2003). The concept of GL is perhaps more useful than GI alone as this relates to the balance of a meal. GL shows how blood glucose levels are determined by quantity of carbohydrate and not just quality.

The impact of food on blood glucose levels is a complex subject and goes beyond GI and GL concepts. Food allergies and intolerance, the balance of gut bacteria, digestive efficiency and adequacy of sulphur needed to initiate and store gastric hormones can potentially influence blood glucose levels. Such discussions are outside of the context of this chapter.

It is possible to choose all 'healthy' foods as components of a meal and still the GL would be high. A breakfast of porridge oats made with water, sweetened with honey, topped with one portion of fresh fruit and a tablespoon of dried fruit, a glass of orange juice and a cup of coffee would have a high GL. Similarly, two slices of wholegrain toast with a thick spread of preserve on each slice, with a fruit juice and cup of coffee would have a high GL.

In comparison, porridge oats made with whole milk, topped with one portion of fresh fruit that is not overly ripe and sprinkled with a tablespoon of mixed nuts and seeds, a juice that is diluted one-third juice to two-thirds water and a coffee would have a significantly lower GL, as would having two eggs on toast, followed by a piece of fresh fruit and a coffee. A strong cup of tea is about equal in caffeine content to a cup of coffee. Green tea and white tea confer similar antioxidant benefits and have substantially lower caffeine content. Withdrawing from caffeine can be problematic, leading to unpleasant symptoms like headaches, irritability and depression. Improving the balance of the diet is a good place to start and drinking tea and coffee as part of a meal, rather than in between, is better as this is less likely to significantly disrupt blood glucose than drinking on its own. Removing tea and coffee from the diet is worth moving toward and *drinking more water*, lessening the strength of tea and coffee and drinking alongside main meals are practical ways of achieving this outcome. Hydration is key for learning, concentration and memory, and it is worth remembering that over 80% of the brain is water (McIlwain and Bachelard, 1985).

Protein: of primary importance

Protein is fundamental for brain function. Amino acids are required to make neurotransmitters. One example is the amino acid tryptophan, which converts to the mood-enhancing neurotransmitter serotonin (useful food sources include fish, turkey, nuts, seeds, bananas and oats). Low serotonin synthesis is associated with depression, fatigue, insomnia, suicide and attention deficit and behavioural disorders (Bralley and Lord, 2001).

Protein is absorbed more slowly than carbohydrates and is therefore less likely to trigger blood sugar fluctuations. Less insulin is likely to be needed as protein meals help to slow down the rate of glucose absorption (Linkner, 2007). Several amino acids are used to make insulin and required to regulate cells involved in maintaining glucose balance (Linkner, 2007).

Fats for life

It has been proposed that the high percentage of omega-3 fats has set apart *Homo sapiens* from other species as, being liquid, they facilitate rapid nerve transmission leading to dexterity and quick thinking. There is substantial evidence emerging that fatty-acid deficiencies may play a part in a wide range of neuro-developmental disorders including ADHD. Evidence that n-3 deficiency may also be an important factor in clinical depression is increasing (Richardson and Puri, 2000).

It is not widely appreciated that the functioning of neurotransmitters and their receptors can be profoundly influenced by the lipid environment (Richardson and Puri, 2000). Omega-3 fats have been shown to be necessary for the proper function of insulin receptors and reduce fasting blood glucose levels (Linkner, 2007). Excess glucose can be converted to triglycerides, and omega-3 fats have been shown to decrease triglyceride levels in cells (Linkner, 2007). Saturated fats (red meat, dairy) are rich sources of triglycerides and have been shown to decrease the ability of insulin to bind at cell receptor sites (Linkner, 2007). Trans fats found in many processed foods behave similarly to saturated fats and are considered more harmful than saturated fats to health (American Heart Association Forums, online).

Oily fish, wholegrain, walnuts, flax, pumpkin seeds and hemp seeds and their oils are excellent sources of omega-3 oils. Both dietary fat and protein in the gut stimulate the release of cholecystokinin, a hormone that plays an important role in the chain of events that lead to satiation and meal termination and could therefore help in appetite suppression (de Graaf *et al*, 2004).

Carbohydrates: sugar and starch and all things 'nice'

In nature, sweet food is generally 'safe'. Our natural desire for sweet food has been exploited since the industrial revolution and particularly so during the latter half of the 20th century. Infant foods and drinks often have added sugar. Professor Yudkin in his book, *Pure, White and Deadly*, republished in 1986, discussed many of the potential damaging effects of sugar that are now being realised. Breast milk is delivered in three distinct phases: protein first, followed by fats and, last, the milk sugar. It is my view that we retain this desire for something sweet at the end of a meal.

Carbohydrates can be simple or complex. Wholegrain, pulses and fibre are good sources of complex carbohydrates and release their sugars slowly. In addition, eating wholegrain provides good levels of B vitamins, chromium, magnesium and zinc, all of which help to maintain blood glucose levels.

Fruit, fruit juice, refined grains and refined sugar are quick-releasing sugars. The fibre from fruit, vegetables, oat and rice bran helps slow down the digestion and absorption of glucose into the bloodstream, prevents excessive secretion of insulin, and improves the uptake of glucose by the liver and other tissues preventing blood glucose levels from remaining high (Murray and Pizzorno, 2000). Eating a whole piece of fruit is therefore better than drinking fruit juice, which has had the fibre removed. A glass of juice could contain the fruit sugar of five or more portions of fruit but we would rarely consume five portions of fruit in one go. Eating fruit at the beginning or end of a meal, or as part of a snack that contains protein and fat, should slow down the absorption of fruit sugar.

Fruit sugar is somewhat better than white sugar as fructose is processed in the liver first before becoming glucose. Most diabetics and hypoglycaemics can tolerate a moderate amount of fructose, but tolerate sucrose poorly. It should be remembered that milk is a 'sweet' fluid as it contains the milk sugar lactose. Low-fat milk will give rise to a higher sugar effect.

OTHER COMMON BLOOD SUGAR DISRUPTERS

- Stimulants, eg. components of tea, coffee, cola and nicotine, can give rise to a release of sugar into the bloodstream. Recent research, albeit on a small sample size, would suggest that avoidance of caffeine could help those with type 2 diabetes (Lane *et al*, 2008).

- Stress initiates the release of sugar into the bloodstream. Stressors include: demanding jobs; redundancy; divorce; separation; loss; pain; toxicity; allergens; stimulants.

- Alcohol consumption interferes with the normal use of glucose in the body, as well as increasing the production of insulin; alcohol can induce reactive hypoglycaemia and sugar cravings (Murray and Pizzorno, 2000).

- Food reactions can disrupt blood glucose balance.

- Physical inactivity has a negative impact on insulin sensitivity.

Worse-case scenario

Described earlier in the chapter were two potential 'healthy' breakfasts that have a high GL. Given a worse-case scenario, this breakfast could be a cereal bowl of refined-sugar-frosted cereal with skimmed milk, fruit cordial, refined bread and jam and coffee with two added teaspoons of sugar. Mid-morning, a can of fizzy drink with a large chocolate bar might be consumed. A can of fizzy drink may contain around seven teaspoons of sugar, and so the day goes on. Besides dietary intake, an average day may have many stressors of all kinds with little physical activity for many people. The day could be a rollercoaster ride of ups and downs in blood sugar balance.

Many people that I have worked with who have mental illness, particularly bipolar depression, have diets like this and many are nicotine dependent. If mental health institutions were able to provide main meals balanced for protein to slow-releasing carbohydrates, include good sources of omega-3 oils, keep patients hydrated and enable physical activity, it is likely that there would be significant mental health benefits. Maintaining improved diet and lifestyle choices in the community is more of a challenge and considerable education and support for mental healthcare workers, carers and the affected individuals are needed to bring about sustainable change.

Response to high blood sugar levels

As mentioned earlier, around five to six grams of glucose in the blood is enough to supply the energy required for body processes that depend on glucose. Imagine 10 or more teaspoons of sugar entering the bloodstream quickly after a fizzy drink and chocolate bar. The body is able to respond and does so for many people day in, day out for many years. For some, many years can go by before real evidence of health problems present themselves. For others, tolerance is less and symptoms manifest sooner. Many people in the population are likely to have problems controlling blood sugar and there are likely to be many undiagnosed diabetics in the population. The long-term complications of diabetes on our physical and mental health are complex and potentially devastating.

Refined sugars enter the bloodstream rapidly, giving rise to an increase in blood sugar. This rise in blood glucose is sensed by the pancreas, which greatly increases its secretion of insulin to drive the blood sugar levels down and can result in symptoms of hypoglycaemia, which include: sweet cravings; need for frequent meals; frequent headaches; dizziness on standing; poor memory and/or concentration; tired shortly after eating; palpitations; feeling shaky; fatigue, particularly in the afternoon; blurred vision; mood swings; depression; anxiety; nervousness; weight gain. Many of these symptoms could indicate other health problems. However, when several symptoms occur and are related to diet and lifestyle, it is reasonable to consider that there is difficulty in maintaining balanced blood sugar levels.

Adrenaline is produced by the adrenal glands in response to the rapid fall in blood sugar levels, which quickly increases the level of glucose in the blood again. Adrenal exhaustion can manifest over time due to the repeated 'insults' and the blood sugar level is not adequately restored. The body can then become insensitive to the action of insulin or the pancreas can also become exhausted. Reactive hypoglycaemia occurs and can lead to diabetes.

Potential impact in the community

Although the association of hypoglycaemia and impaired mental function is accepted, the role of hypoglycaemia in various psychological disorders is less well understood. Aggressive and criminal behaviour has been linked to hypoglycaemia as shown in controlled studies with psychiatric patients and habitually violent and impulsive criminals. Aggressive behaviour is a known symptom associated with hypoglycaemia in insulin-dependent diabetics. It is unfortunate that testing for reactive hypoglycaemia is not more commonly performed in depressed or anxious individuals or those expressing behavioural problems.

Refined carbohydrates and starches in the multi-forms (bread, cereals, pasta and potatoes) are generally cheap fuels compared with protein-rich food. Beans and lentils are also relatively cheap food but not commonly consumed other than as baked beans, which often have sugar added. Beans and lentils contain good levels of fibre and nutrients that help to balance blood sugar levels.

The psychological and practical impact for individuals and families on low incomes to make a shift towards more complex carbohydrates and protein-rich food is significant. Sugars and fats have what is called the organoleptic appeal, ie. they have the taste-good factor. The psychological impact of changing to a basic diet of wholegrain, beans and lentils for an individual or family who are already feeling deprived, may prove insurmountable, particularly with the impact of supermarkets, television and the rest of the media. In order to break the cycle of cravings for sweet food and stimulants, it can be appreciated just how important coaching skills are for health professionals giving out advice.

In clinical practice, I find that the most important nutritional intervention is to manage the GL of each meal and snack using healthy foods and drinks.

BREAKFAST

- 1/3 mug of porridge oats and 1/2 mug of (preferably organic) full-fat cow or goat milk or soy milk plus 1/2 mug of water with one dessertspoon of mixed, ground flax, pumpkin and hemp seeds or a small handful of walnuts over cooked porridge and one firm banana.

- Two poached, boiled or scrambled eggs on wholegrain toast (preferably rye) with grilled tomatoes and grilled mushrooms.

LUNCH/DINNER

- Palm-size portion of fish, poultry or meat or two eggs or 1/2 pack of tofu with different colour vegetables equal in amount to eating two to three medium apples. Salad, soup, baked, steamed, stir-fried or grilled vegetables. Add one dessertspoon of omega-3, -6 and -9 oil over salad or over vegetables once cooked. Use herbs and spices to flavour. A little Tamari soy sauce adds flavour to tofu and cooked vegetables.

- 1/2 mug of cooked beans or lentils with one cup of cooked rice or wholegrain pasta or other wholegrain with two to three vegetable portions. Flavour with herbs and spices.

- Beans on wholegrain toast with salad makes a quick and economic meal.

- Bean or lentil soup with wholegrain bread is another simple option.

SNACKS

- Small handful of nuts and seeds and a crisp apple.

- 30 g of cheese and a raw carrot or peppers or celery.

- Two crackers with a tablespoon of hummus or hazelnut, almond or cashew nut butter on each cracker.

- Small pot of plain yoghurt with a fresh piece of fruit or stir in one tablespoon of nut or seed butter.

DRINKS

- 6 x 250 ml glasses of quality water daily.

- One cup of tea, if desired, after a meal.

- 2–3 mugs of other green tea, white tea, rooibos, peppermint, fennel or other herbal or fruit teas.

- Barley Cup or Yannoh are good coffee alternatives.

- One cup of coffee, only if needed, after breakfast or lunch and preferably avoid.

- One glass of red wine with lunch or dinner, only if needed, and preferably avoid.

Nutritional supplements

As the name implies, nutritional supplements are supplementary to the diet and lifestyle of the individual. They should not be considered alternatives to a balanced diet. It is impossible to emulate the myriad of plant compounds and nutrients that naturally occur in food in a supplement. Nevertheless, the addition of a multivitamin mineral, providing at least 100% of the recommended nutrient intake, should help to bridge the gap in the diet or lend some support for increased requirements placed on the body as a result of modern living.

Several nutrients and compounds have been identified in research studies as potentially helpful for managing blood sugar levels. Many studies are conducted in diabetic or hypoglycaemic individuals and many are animal studies. In combination with a balanced diet and modifications to lifestyle, the following supplements could be of help. Dosage in clinical practice is considered on a one-to-one basis and often after laboratory testing for nutrient status and adjusted accordingly with ongoing monitoring.

For many of the nutrients or compounds discussed opposite a dosage or dosage range has been included and would be best used under the guidance of a nutritional therapist who is trained to use therapeutic levels of nutritional supplements. Supplementing individual nutrients and compounds can imbalance other nutrients. Several botanicals have also been shown to help blood sugar balance but have not been discussed here.

Supplement	Mechanism of action	Dosage
Alpha lipoic acid	Improves insulin sensitivity, decreases glucose and insulin levels, improves glucose uptake, antioxidant	200–1,000 mg (Linkner, 2007)
Antioxidants (vitamins A, C, E, zinc and selenium are among the better known antioxidants)	Defends against oxidative stress, which can increase sugar levels and impair insulin secretion (Linkner, 2007)	
Biotin	Improves insulin sensitivity, reduces insulin requirements in type 1 diabetics (Kelly, 2000)	
Chromium	Aids insulin in increasing uptake of glucose into cells, shown to reduce body weight, increase lean body mass and improve mood	At least 200 mcg day for 'optimal' blood glucose control (Murray and Pizzorno, 2000)
Cinnamon	Has generally been considered supportive to blood sugar control in diabetics, but a recent meta-analysis found no significant benefits on fasting blood glucose, lipids or glycosylated haemoglobin	Toxicity concerns regarding consistent intake of high doses of whole cinnamon (Linkner, 2007)
Magnesium	Activates glucose transport and insulin mediated glucose uptake	Dosage 200–800 mg daily (Linkner, 2007)
Manganese	Required for many enzymes involved in blood sugar control (Murray and Pizzorno, 2000)	
Potassium	Improves insulin sensitivity and insulin secretion (Murray and Pizzorno, 2000)	Caution is needed in supplementing potassium in diabetic patients as renal handling of potassium can be impaired
Vanadium	Improves insulin receptivity and helps regulate fasting blood sugar levels (Boden et al, 1996)	
Vitamin B1 (thiamine)	A co-factor in carbohydrate metabolism and associated with reduced glycosylation of proteins (Evans et al, 2003)	

cont. ▷

Supplement	Mechanism of action	Dosage
Vitamin B3 (niacin)	Works with chromium, aiding insulin in increasing uptake of glucose into cells. Thought to help restore beta cell function or slow down their destruction. Can disrupt blood sugar control in some diabetics and so monitoring is required	Niacin as inositol hexaniacinate is considered a safer form and is reported to give slightly better results than standard niacin. 600–1,800 mg daily as inositol hexaniacinate – no adverse reactions in 153 patients (Murray and Pizzorno, 2000)
Vitamin B6 (pyridoxine)	Shown to help prevent glycosylation of proteins (Solomon and Cohen, 1989). B6 is also required for the synthesis of insulin	
Vitamin C	Shown to reduce glucose levels, glycosylated haemoglobin, insulin resistance and LDL cholesterol. Also shown to increase HDL cholesterol	One to two grams daily for influence on cholesterol (Linkner, 2007)
Vitamin E	High dosage has been shown to improve the action of insulin. Conflicting data, and one study showed that insulin status was made worse in some patients (Kelly, 2000)	A four-week, double-blind, randomised trial showed benefit in supplementing 600 mg of vitamin E daily in insulin-sensitive hypertensive patients (Barbagallo et al, 1999). 900 international units of vitamin E has been shown to improve insulin sensitivity (Murray and Pizzorno, 2000)
Zinc	Plays a clear role in the synthesis, storage and secretion of insulin. Zinc has been shown to help protect against the destruction of beta cells	Dosage 30 mg a day in diabetics (Murray and Pizzorno, 2000)

References

American Heart Association Forums (2007). Available at: http://my.americanheart.org/ jiveforum/thread.jspa?messageID=41131 [accessed 14/07/08].

Barbagallo M, Dominguez LJ, Tagliamonte MR, Resnick LM and Paolisso G (1999) Effects of vitamin E and glutathione on glucose metabolism: role of magnesium. *Hypertension* **34** (4) 1002–1006.

Barker D (1994) The foetal origins of adult disease. *Proceedings of the Royal Society of London* **262** (1363) 37–43.

Bland J and Jones D (2006) Clinical approaches to hormonal and neuroendocrine imbalances. In: *Textbook of Functional Medicine* (p618). Gig Harbor: The Institute for Functional Medicine.

Boden G, Chen X, Ruiz J, van Rossum GDV and Turco Sl (1996) Effects of vanadyl sulphate on carbohydrate and lipid metabolism in patients with non-insulin-dependent diabetes mellitus. *Metabolism* **45** (9) 1130–1135.

Bralley J and Lord R (2001) *Laboratory Evaluations in Molecular Medicine* (p193). Norcross: IAMM.

Brand-Miller JC, Thomas M, Swan V, Ahmad ZI, Petocz P and Colagiuri S (2003) Physiological validation of the concept of glycemic load in lean young adults. *Journal of Nutrition* **133** (9) 2728–2732.

Evans JL, Goldfine ID, Maddux BA and Grodsky GM (2003) Are oxidative stress-activated signalling pathways mediators of insulin resistance and beta-cell dysfunction? *Diabetes* **52** (1) 1–8.

de Graaf C, Blom WAM, Smeets PAM, Stafleu A and Hendriks HFJ (2004) Biomarkers of satiation and satiety. *American Journal of Clinical Nutrition* **79** (6) 946–961.

Jenkins DJ, Wolever TM, Taylor RH, Barker H, Fielden H, Baldwin JM, Bowling AC, Newman HC, Jenkins AL and Goff DV (1981) Glycemic index of foods: a physiological basis for carbohydrate exchange. *American Journal of Clinical Nutrition* **34** (3) 362–366.

Kelly G (2000) Insulin resistance: lifestyle and nutritional interventions. *Alternative Medicine Review* **5** (2) 109–132.

Lane JD, Feinglos MN and Surwit RS (2008) Caffeine increases ambulatory glucose and postprandial responses in coffee drinkers with type 2 diabetes. *Diabetes Care* **31** (2) 221–222.

Linkner E (2007) Insulin resistance and the metabolic syndrome. In: D Rakel (2007) *Integrative Medicine* (2nd edition). Philadelphia: Saunders Elsevier.

McIlwain H and Bachelard HS (1985) *Biochemistry and the Central Nervous System.* Edinburgh: Churchill Livingstone.

Murray T and Pizzorno J (2000) *Textbook of Natural Medicine* (2nd edition). New York: Churchill Livingstone.

Richardson A and Puri B (2000) The potential role of fatty acids in ADHD. *The Nutrition Practitioner* **2** (2) 15–21.

Solomon LR and Cohen K (1989) Erythrocyte O2 transport and metabolism and effects of vitamin B6 therapy in type II diabetes mellitus. *Diabetes* **38** (7) 881–886.

Yudkin JS (1986) *Pure, White and Deadly.* London: Viking.

Chapter 12
Nutritional approaches to the management of eating disorders and eating distress

JANE NODDER

Eating disorders are complex psychological conditions characterised by *'a definite disturbance of eating habits or weight-control behaviour'* (Fairburn and Harrison, 2003) and *'distress or excessive concern about body shape or body weight'* (Becker *et al*, 1999). Eating disorders have a wide range of symptoms and contributing factors, and frequent overlap.

The fourth edition of the *Diagnostic and Statistical Manual of Mental Disorders* (DSM-IV) of the American Psychiatric Association (1994), identifies three specific disorders: anorexia nervosa and bulimia nervosa (probably the best known of the conditions) and *'eating disorder not otherwise specified'* (EDNOS, or *'atypical eating disorder'* in the UK) (American Psychiatric Association, 1994). EDNOS describes *'eating disorders of clinical severity that do not conform to the diagnostic criteria for anorexia nervosa or bulimia nervosa'* and includes binge eating disorder (BED) (Fairburn and Harrison, 2003).

In clinical practice, EDNOS may be as common as anorexia and bulimia nervosa (Millar, 1998; Ricca *et al*, 2001; Turner and Bryant-Waught, 2004) and in the absence of recovery these conditions may themselves evolve into anorexia or bulimia nervosa (Fairburn and Harrison, 2003). Obesity does not appear in the DSM-IV as it is not always associated with a psychological or behavioural syndrome (American Psychiatric Association, 1994).

RISK FACTORS ASSOCIATED WITH EATING DISORDERS

- Female gender
- Perfectionist, rigid, risk-avoidant personality traits
- Dieting
- History of obesity or family history of obesity
- History of an eating disorder and/or family history of an eating disorder
- Personal or family history of drug and/or alcohol abuse
- Personal or family history of depression
- Elite performance (male and female)
- Personal or family history of physical or sexual abuse, teasing and harassment

Source: Harvard Eating Disorders Center (2006–2008, online)

Nutritional approaches to eating disorders – a brief history

Although treatment for eating disorders primarily focuses on psychological approaches, there is evidence for addressing their nutrition-related aspects in recovery. Herrin (2003) describes how, back in 1694, a patient presumed to have anorexia nervosa was advised to use a *'milk diet'*, and, in 1768, a patient was *'prevailed upon by her physician to take more nourishing food, to increase the quantity daily'*. During the early 20th century, anorexia nervosa was considered firstly a *'purely psychological disorder'* and then an *'endocrine disorder'*, but, by the 1940s, psychological treatment approaches were supported by advice on a 'proper diet'. In 1950, Ancel Keys showed how under-nutrition interferes directly with cognitive and emotional function providing support for nutrition approaches in the treatment of eating disorders (Keys *et al*, 1950).

Early in her career, the psychiatrist Hilde Bruch argued that *'efforts to restore weight were only beneficial if they were part of an integrated treatment programme focused mainly on correcting underlying psychological and family problems'* (Silverman, 1997). Later, Bruch concluded that *'nutritional restitution (was) a pre-requisite for psychotherapy to be effective'* (Bruch, 1985).

During the 1990s, both the American Psychiatric Association (APA) and the American Dietetic Association (ADA) recognised nutrition counselling as an essential component in eating disorder treatment alongside psychosocial and medical interventions. In its most recent position paper, the ADA restated *'that nutrition intervention, including nutritional counselling, by a registered dietician (RD) is an essential component of the team treatment of patients with anorexia nervosa, bulimia nervosa, and other eating disorders'* (American Dietetic Association, 2006). In the UK, the Eating Disorders, Special Interest Group (EDSIG) of the Royal College of Psychiatrists has produced *Guidelines for the Nutritional Management of Anorexia Nervosa* (Winston *et al*, 2004), and in 2004 the National Institute for Clinical Excellence (NICE) published a clinical guideline for managing eating disorders, which includes recommendations for nutritional approaches.

DIAGNOSTIC CRITERIA FOR ANOREXIA NERVOSA

- Refusal to maintain body weight at or above a minimally normal weight for age and height (eg. weight loss leading to maintenance of body weight less than 85% of that expected, or failure to make expected weight gain during period of growth, leading to body weight less than 85% of that expected)*.

- Intense fear of gaining weight or becoming fat, even though underweight.

- Disturbance in the way in which one's body weight or shape is experienced, undue influence of body weight or shape on self-evaluation, or denial of the seriousness of the current low body weight.

- In postmenarcheal females** amenorrhoea, ie. the absence of at least three consecutive menstrual cycles. (A woman is considered to have amenorrhoea if her periods occur only following hormone, eg. oestrogen, administration.) cont. ▷

Specify type

- **Restricting type:** during the current episode of anorexia nervosa, the person has not regularly engaged in binge eating or purging behaviour (ie. self-induced vomiting or the misuse of laxatives, diuretics or enemas).

- **Binge-eating/purging type:** during the current episode of anorexia nervosa, the person has regularly engaged in binge eating or purging behaviour (ie. self-induced vomiting or the misuse of laxatives, diuretics or enemas).

* Many experts use body mass index (BMI) below 17.5 – calculated as weight in kilograms divided by height in metres squared – as a diagnostic tool for anorexia.
** In men, endocrine disturbance manifests as loss of sexual interest and potency.

Source: American Psychiatric Association (1994) in Garfinkel (2002)

DIAGNOSTIC CRITERIA FOR BULIMIA NERVOSA

- Recurrent episodes of binge eating. An episode of binge eating is characterised by both of the following:

  - eating, in a discrete period of time (eg. within any two-hour period), an amount of food that is definitely larger than most people would eat during a similar period of time and under similar circumstances

  - a sense of lack of control over eating during the episode (eg. a feeling that one cannot stop eating or control what or how much one is eating).

- Recurrent inappropriate compensatory behaviour in order to prevent weight gain, such as self-induced vomiting, misuse of laxatives, diuretics, enemas, or other medication, fasting or excessive exercise.

- The binge eating and inappropriate compensatory behaviours both occur, on average, at least twice a week for three months.

- Self-evaluation is unduly influenced by body shape and weight.

- The disturbance does not occur exclusively during episodes of anorexia nervosa.

Specify type

- **Purging type:** during the current episode of bulimia nervosa, the person has regularly engaged in self-induced vomiting or the misuse of laxatives, diuretics or enemas.

- **Non-purging type:** during the current episode of bulimia nervosa, the person has used other inappropriate compensatory behaviours, such as fasting or excessive exercise, but has not regularly engaged in self-induced vomiting or the misuse of laxatives, diuretics or enemas.

Source: American Psychiatric Association (1994) in Garfinkel (2002)

RESEARCH CRITERIA FOR BINGE EATING DISORDER

- Recurrent episodes of binge eating. An episode of binge eating is characterised by both of the following:

  - eating, in a discrete period of time (eg. within any two-hour period), an amount of food that is definitely larger than most people would eat in a similar period of time under similar circumstances

  - a sense of lack of control over eating during the episode (eg. a feeling that one cannot stop eating or control what or how much one is eating).

- The binge eating episodes are associated with at least three of the following:

  - eating much more rapidly than normal

  - eating until feeling uncomfortably full

  - eating large amounts of food when not feeling physically hungry

  - eating alone because of being embarrassed by how much one is eating

  - feeling disgusted with oneself, depressed or feeling very guilty after overeating.

- Marked distress regarding binge eating.

- The binge eating occurs, on average, at least two days a week for six months.

- The binge eating is not associated with the regular use of inappropriate compensatory behaviours (eg. purging, fasting, excessive exercise) and does not occur exclusively during the course of anorexia nervosa or bulimia nervosa.

Source: American Psychiatric Association (1994) in Garfinkel (2002)

Possible biochemical imbalances in eating disorders

Eating disorders can have a major effect on physical and mental health through altered nutritional status due to starvation, binge eating, purging and erratic eating patterns (Rome and Ammerman, 2003). Dieting, skipping meals and binge eating food that is high in sugar and refined carbohydrates may disrupt blood glucose mechanisms leading to low blood sugar levels, cravings and desensitisation of cells to insulin (Johnson *et al*, 1994).

Serotonin metabolism and neurotransmitter balance may also be disturbed. When neurotransmitters are present in sufficient amounts, mood and emotions are stable. If they are depleted, individuals may starve or overeat to try and manage mood (Wurtman and Wurtman, 1996). Serotonin plays a role in controlling carbohydrate intake, promoting sleep and regulating impulsive and obsessional behaviours (Kaye, 2007). It is produced from the amino acid tryptophan in the presence of insulin, vitamin B6 and zinc (Kaye and Weltzin, 1991). Dieting has been shown to deplete levels of tryptophan very quickly, particularly in women (Cowen *et al*, 1996; Wolfe *et al*, 1997).

There may be a link between low serotonin and some of the symptoms that commonly characterise bulimia nervosa, eg. depression, impulsivity, irritability and emotional volatility (Weltzin *et al*, 1995), although it is not clear if low serotonin levels are a cause or result of bulimia nervosa (Weltzin *et al*, 1995). Vomiting suppresses serotonin levels as the body loses the essential nutrients required for serotonin production and altered serotonin function may persist even after recovery from anorexia and bulimia nervosa (Bailer *et al*, 2005; 2007; Kaye, 2007).

Some eating disorder patients describe an 'addictive' relationship with certain foods. They report strong cravings for these foods to get a 'lift', and/or withdrawal symptoms if they reduce consumption of a food they regularly consume (Wurtman and Wurtman, 1996; Pelchat, 2002). Incomplete digestion of proteins, such as casein and gluten, may stimulate the production of opioid peptides that can contribute to an 'addictive' sensation and result in food cravings (Mercer and Holder, 1997). The consumption of highly palatable sweet foods and alcohol can also stimulate endogenous opioid peptide activity and promote analgesia, possibly reinforcing an individual's preference for such foods (Drewnowski *et al*, 1992; Mercer and Holder, 1997).

Sugar may affect neurotransmitters such as serotonin and dopamine and the release of endorphins. Colantuoni *et al* (2002) demonstrated that rats tended to binge eat when given food and sugar-water after food deprivation for 12 hours. In addition, the rats responded to the sugar in a way that was similar to their response to drugs like heroin and cocaine, and showed signs of withdrawal-like anxiety when researchers blocked their brains' opioid system. Volkow *et al* (2002) demonstrated that just the sight or smell of food can spike levels of the neurotransmitter dopamine even if the study subjects did not eat the food and, hence, had no pleasure associated with it.

The gastrointestinal (GI) effects of starvation and binge eating include delayed gastric emptying and disturbances in GI motility, resulting in symptoms such as constipation, early satiety and bloating (Rome and Ammerman, 2003). There may also be disturbances in satiety mechanisms normally controlled by cholecystokinin (CCK), grelin, neuropeptide Y (NpY), serotonin, leptin and endorphins (National Institute for Clinical Excellence, 2004) secondary to disturbed eating patterns and weight loss (Fairburn and Harrison, 2003).

Amenorrhoea (absence of menstruation) is the main manifestation of sex hormone imbalance in anorexia nervosa (Rome and Ammerman, 2003). The presence of amenorrhoea reduces the prevalence of anaemia in anorexia nervosa, although vegetarian patients may have microcytic anaemia (Rome and Ammerman, 2003). Low oestrogen status has been linked to bulimia nervosa (Naessén, 2007), and oligomenorrhoea or amenorrhoea can occur in bulimic patients of normal weight (Pirke *et al*, 1986). Other endocrine imbalances include hypercortisolaemia with osteopenia in anorexia nervosa, and thyroid abnormalities, such as a reduction in triiodothyronine (T3) and thyoxine (T4) levels and an increase in reverse T3 (O'Connor *et al*, 2000; Rome and Ammerman, 2003). Essential fatty acids (omega-6 and omega-3) are needed for the production of sex and stress hormones and neurotransmitters, and for metabolic function. Low fat diets have been associated with endocrine disruption and depression (Bruinsma and Taren, 2000; Logan, 2003) and eating disorder patients frequently avoid fat in their diet.

ABNORMALITIES THAT MAY INDICATE AN UNDISCLOSED EATING DISORDER

Somatic	Behavioural
Arrested growth	Change in eating habits
Marked change or frequent fluctuation in weight	Difficulty eating in social situations
Inability to gain weight	Reluctance to be weighed
Fatigue	Depression
Constipation or diarrhoea	Social withdrawal
Susceptibility to fractures	Absence from school or work
Delayed menarche	Deceptive or secretive behaviour
Hypokalemia, hyperphosphatemia	Stealing (eg. to obtain food)
Metabolic acidosis or alkalosis	Substance abuse
High serum amylase levels	Excessive exercise

Source: Becker *et al* (1999)

Aim of nutritional approaches for eating disorders

Although psychological approaches are the foundation for eating disorder treatment, the medical complexity of the conditions demands a collaborative approach from a mixed discipline team of psychological, nutritional and medical experts working closely together (Becker *et al*, 1999; Herrin, 1999; American Dietetic Association, 2006). Treatment approaches are designed to stabilise medical and nutritional status and identify and resolve psychosocial concerns (Becker *et al*, 1999; American Dietetic Association, 2006). Many of the physical signs and symptoms of eating disorders can be reversed by nutrition rehabilitation, with the possible exception of reduced bone density (Fairburn and Harrison, 2003; Golden and Meyer, 2004).

Practitioners working with nutritional approaches to eating disorders or disordered eating must have appropriate skills, training and experience, including specific knowledge of nutrition and sound training in nutritional assessment and counselling. They must know how to:

■ provide accurate information about the role of nutrients in addressing the physical and psychological effects of binge eating, starving and purging and in rebalancing physiology and biochemistry (McFarland, 1995)

■ teach patients about energy balance, body weight regulation and the physical consequences of starvation and purging behaviours. Normalising eating makes binge eating less likely and helps to stop purging (American Dietetic Association, 2006)

■ support the patient in changing their behaviour around food including encouraging any necessary weight gain and maintenance and discouraging dieting and compulsive weighing (Herrin, 2003; Golden and Meyer, 2004; American Dietetic Association, 2006)

■ address concerns that the patient may have regarding long-term consequences, such as osteoporosis (Mehler, 2003), amenorrhoea, infertility and other endocrine disorders (Bruinsma and Taren, 2000) and obesity (Kaplan and Cliska, 1999)

■ address lifestyle issues such as exercise and stress management and support the delivery of psychological treatments and the use of any medication (American Dietetic Association, 2006).

Practitioners should be familiar with inpatient treatment approaches and have some knowledge of methodologies, such as motivational interviewing and cognitive behavioural therapy. They must be clear about their personal and professional boundaries and know when to seek additional help and how to ensure appropriate medical monitoring for a patient (Herrin, 2003). They also need to understand their personal relationship with, and attitude to, food. Nutrition professionals should encourage patients to share significant 'non-nutrition' issues with their psychology professional, and arrange for their work with nutrition to be formally supervised by an experienced psychotherapist (Herrin, 2003).

QUESTIONS A PRACTITIONER MIGHT ASK TO CLARIFY CONCERNS OR SUSPICIONS ABOUT A POSSIBLE EATING DISORDER

■ What does normal healthy eating mean to you?

■ How do you know when you are physically hungry?

■ How would you describe your current relationship with food?

■ Do you regularly turn to food when you have a problem to solve?

■ How much time do you spend each day thinking about food, your weight and exercise?

■ Are you preoccupied with food and your next opportunity to eat?

■ Have you ever felt ashamed after eating certain foods?

cont. ▷

- Have you ever eaten large amounts of food in a short space of time?

- Are you always 'on or off' a diet or about to 'start again' tomorrow?

- Do you avoid certain foods or carry lists of 'forbidden' foods in your head?

- Does it concern you if others see what, how much or how often you eat?

- Do you eat in secret?

- Have you ever made yourself sick, taken laxatives/diuretics or fasted after eating a large quantity of food?

- Would you describe yourself as 'in control' of food and your eating?

- How often do you weigh yourself?

- Do you think you have an eating disorder?

Overall nutritional strategy for eating disorders and disordered eating

Eating disorder patients frequently claim to be experts in nutrition, although much of their knowledge may be incorrect or misconceived (Fairburn and Hill, 2005). The first steps in nutritional management are to obtain a detailed dietary history and to fully explore and understand the patient's eating behaviours and their knowledge and attitudes with regard to food (Golden and Meyer, 2004). Treatment can then be focused on structuring eating patterns to encourage three small meals with two/three snacks, or four/five small meals, at three to four hour intervals throughout the day. To reduce anxiety and binge eating, stabilise or maintain body weight or bring about a slow reduction in weight if necessary, food plans should be balanced for the major food groups and based on 1,500–2,500 calories as appropriate for the individual patient. It is useful to aim for 45–55% of calories from carbohydrate, 20–25% from protein and 25–30% from fat (Willard *et al*, 1983; Herrin, 2003).

Depending on the patient's size and weight, each meal should include 20–30 g of protein containing all essential amino acids to help reduce cravings for refined carbohydrates (Rolls *et al*, 1988). Including foods high in the amino acid tryptophan (eg. milk, poultry, eggs, red meats, soybeans, tofu and almonds) may help to support serotonin production.

Eating a wide range of vegetables and two to three servings of fruit per day provides carbohydrate, fibre and essential vitamins, minerals and phytonutrients for metabolic function. Food plans should include up to 1,500 mg per day of calcium from foods, such as dairy products, green leafy vegetables, soya products and canned fish, and supplements (Herrin, 2003).

Daily intake of essential omega fatty acids from oily fish, nuts and seeds can support neurotransmitter function and help with symptoms of low mood and depression and hormone balance (Herrin, 1999).

Adequate water intake is important. Under-eating, vomiting and laxative use all result in dehydration followed by water retention. This may be experienced by some patients as weight gain leading to further purging or dieting (Garner, 1997). Some patients may 'water load' to blunt appetite, increase weight, initiate vomiting or eliminate 'toxins' (Rome and Ammerman, 2003).

Reducing sugars, refined products and stimulants, such as coffee, can support blood glucose control, insulin output and mood (Brand Miller *et al*, 1997; Frost and Dornhorst, 2000). However, for bulimics and binge eaters in particular, placing such foods 'off limits' can make them more desirable and raise fears in the patient that they will eventually binge on the very foods they are continuing to deny themselves. Including some 'fun food' as part of the daily food plan can make such foods less 'desirable' or 'forbidden' (Herrin, 2003). As they progress, patients can gradually be encouraged to include foods previously labelled as 'forbidden' or 'binge' foods.

Practical implementation of nutritional approaches

Nutrition counselling sessions would probably start on a weekly basis and move to fortnightly or monthly depending on the patient's progress. When working with a patient it can be helpful to start with their current pattern, making gradual, but steady, changes at each visit to normalise food intake without creating unnecessary anxiety. Any food plan must protect against under- and over-eating and recognise that it can be difficult to meet basic nutrient needs below 1,500 calories per day (Sizer and Whitney, 2000; Golden and Meyer, 2004). In addition, under-nutrition often results in cognitive deficits, which may limit the efficacy of psychotherapy (Bruch, 1985).

Nutritional approaches are often more successful when the patient plays an active role in food planning and decisions (Brand Miller *et al*, 1997). Patients should leave each counselling session with a realistic goal to work on (eg. eating breakfast, adding an afternoon snack), and be encouraged to keep full records of food intake (Golden and Meyer, 2004), linked to mood/emotions/situations between sessions. This record can be reviewed at subsequent visits.

Nutrition professionals can helpfully explain to patients that many of their symptoms may be due to the eating disorder itself, and that they are likely to resolve once consistent eating patterns are established. They can also identify nutritional interventions to help manage symptoms, such as constipation, and deal with any side effects from eliminating binge eating and purging behaviours.

Issues in the early stages of treatment

Recovery can be slow and requires considerable commitment of time and energy from all involved. Patients often struggle with resistance and ambivalence, so goals should be small and achievable. Practitioners should know how to deal with a number of issues that are common in the early stages of treatment. These include:

■ encouraging patients recovering from anorexia nervosa to increase their food intake for a sustained period of time and to maintain the weight they have gained

■ eliminating purging or other compensatory behaviours in bulimic patients, before working to identify binge trigger foods and establish a structured eating pattern

■ helping patients with bulimia nervosa or binge eating disorder to understand the mechanics of weight control and the effects of binge eating on metabolism – bulimics/binge eaters who are overweight may want to lose weight long before their eating is actually stable (Fairburn and Hill, 2005)

■ increasing macronutrient intake (particularly fats and carbohydrates) over time and at a pace that does not create unnecessary anxiety

■ supporting the patient in making choices that legalise all foods so that nothing is 'forbidden' or labelled as 'bad' or 'fattening'

■ discouraging patients with regard to dieting and inappropriate weighing.

Moving the patient on nutritionally

As the patient recovers, the nutritional programme can be 'fine-tuned' to manage any remaining biochemical imbalances (eg. thyroid function or gastrointestinal symptoms) that may be impacting on progress. Identifying when to start such action can be difficult; early intervention to correct specific physiological imbalances may have a poorer outcome if the client is still binge eating, starving or purging, but improving overall nutrient status per se, may, in itself, resolve certain imbalances and symptoms. Specialist help from an experienced nutrition professional could be appropriate at this stage in the recovery process.

Supplementation and eating disorders

Supplementation with vitamins and minerals may be used by clinicians treating patients with eating disorders because:

■ it can be difficult to satisfy nutrient needs on diets that provide less than 1,500 calories a day (Schebendach and Nussbaum, 1992)

■ higher-calorie diets may not, in themselves, provide the level of nutrients needed during weight restoration in anorexia nervosa (Schebendach and Nussbaum, 1992)

■ the type of food eaten in binges is often devoid of vitamins and minerals (Herrin, 2003).

Despite the fact that some vitamins and minerals (eg. zinc) have come under close scrutiny for the treatment of eating disorders, there is little evidence to support their extensive use with eating disorder patients. Studies on individual nutrients are generally experimental and small, and the administration of single supplements is not recommended (NICE, 2004). Specific vitamin and mineral deficiencies can usually be remedied by restoring normal nutrition or the temporary use of multivitamin and mineral supplements until dietary intake is adequate (Golden and Meyer, 2004; NICE, 2004).

The use of supplements with eating disorder patients must take account of medication, purging behaviours, the compromised physical condition of the patient and views of others in the treatment team. Any prescription should be given by an experienced nutrition professional. Multivitamin and mineral formulations should not contain more than 100% of the RDA for any vitamin or mineral with the exception of calcium intake, which should reach a total maximum (food and supplements) of 1,500 mg per day (Herrin, 2003). It is important to remind patients that supplements do not contain macronutrients and are not a replacement for improving food and calorie intake. Self-prescription should be discouraged to avoid combinations of supplements that may give rise to toxicity issues.

Where supplements are prescribed, it is important to eliminate purging behaviours to allow for appropriate absorption, and it may be useful to consider using powders or sub-lingual forms for patients with sore mouths and throats due to purging. Good-quality supplemental foods, such as sports bars and energy drinks, may be helpful for short-term use.

Working with specific populations and situations
Working in the community or private practice

Practitioners working with nutritional approaches for eating disorders should always be part of a wider, multidisciplinary treatment team that includes a health professional responsible for medical monitoring. A member of the treatment team should also hold responsibility for regular weight monitoring and this aspect of treatment should be discussed clearly with the patient (Golden and Meyer, 2004).

When assessing patients for treatment, practitioners *must* be certain that any weight loss has been adequately restored and that eating patterns and food intake are stable. Inpatient care should be considered where weight is very unstable or extremely low, if there are serious physical complications, for example, severe electrolyte imbalances, cardiac disturbances, other acute medical disorders or behavioural issues, such as treatment-resistant bingeing, severe or intractable vomiting or laxative use, risk of psychosis or suicide, or any other symptoms that are not responding to outpatient treatment (Anderson *et al*, 1990). Refeeding of very low-weight patients is a highly skilled procedure requiring specialist knowledge and close monitoring to reduce the risk of 'refeeding syndrome' (McFarland, 1995).

Food allergies/intolerances, elimination diets and eating disorders

Practitioners must be aware of the particular issues involved in elimination diets and eating disorders. Patients may claim that their gastrointestinal symptoms are the result of food intolerances. However, this presentation can be part of the pathology of their disorder and may be used to exclude certain food groups from the diet. While classic food allergies, such as to peanuts, other nuts, shellfish etc, are potentially life-threatening conditions requiring medical supervision and elimination of culprit foods from an individual's diet for life, any other elimination approach must be used with the greatest caution in patients with eating disorders or disordered eating patterns. Patients in this population need a nutrient-dense diet from a wide variety of foods, and food groups should only be limited where it is very clear that eating particular foods is substantially blocking recovery. Alternatives must always be found to ensure that necessary nutrient and energy needs are met in patients who believe they have food intolerances (Herrin, 2003). Always seek advice from a dietician or nutrition professional with appropriate experience in this field.

Vegetarians and vegans

Vegetarianism is more common in people with eating disorders (particularly anorexia nervosa) and may justifiably be considered part of the psychopathology when it develops alongside the eating disorder (Gilbody *et al*, 1999; Sullivan and Damani, 2000). It is important to ensure that vegetarian choices are for reasons other than being able to avoid foods seen as high in fat or calories, and to check that adequate amounts of protein, calcium, iron, zinc and vitamin B12 are available in the diet (Draper *et al*, 1993; Janelle and Barr, 1995). Vegan diets probably present an unacceptable level of risk (particularly with regard to anorexia nervosa) (Winston *et al*, 2004). In general, religious dietary restrictions should be respected unless they present a serious threat to recovery or represent a considerable part of the patient's pathology (Winston *et al*, 2004).

Male patients, children and adolescents

There are no particular marked differences in terms of the aetiology of eating disorders among men, and no indication that special techniques are needed for the treatment of male patients (Anderson, 2002).

The goals for working with children and adolescents with eating disorders are similar to those for working with adults. However, the specific nutritional needs of growth and development of these patients indicate that their management should be the responsibility of professionals experienced in working with this population and must involve parents (or caregivers) (NICE, 2004). Young athletes, particularly females, are particularly at risk of developing the 'female athlete triangle' of disordered eating, amenorrhoea and osteopenia (Curry and Jaffe, 1998; Rome and Ammerman, 2003).

Co-morbid/co-existent conditions

Practitioners working with eating disorders and co-morbid/co-existent conditions (eg. substance abuse, diabetes, coeliac disease, pregnancy and lactation, Crohn's disease, obesity) must be skilled in the nutritional management of both conditions. Again, they should work as part of a team of qualified health professionals to meet the patient's treatment goals.

Conclusion

Eating disorders are complex mental health conditions with potentially serious complications and care must include psychological treatments, regular medical monitoring, and possibly medication (Becker *et al*, 1999). Although nutritional counselling should not be offered as a sole treatment for eating disorders (NICE, 2004), by addressing food intake, eating behaviours and biochemical imbalances, suitably qualified practitioners can, in collaboration with other specialists, support patients in recovery.

References

American Dietetic Association (2006) Position of the American Dietetic Association: nutrition intervention in the treatment of anorexia nervosa, bulimia nervosa, and other eating disorders. *Journal of the American Dietetic Association* **106** (12) 2073–2082.

American Psychiatric Association (1994) *Diagnostic and Statistical Manual of Mental Disorders* (4th edition). Washington: American Psychiatric Association.

Anderson AE (2002) Eating disorders in males. In: KD Brownell and CG Fairburn (Eds) *Eating Disorders and Obesity: A comprehensive handbook* (2nd edition). New York: Guilford Press.

Anderson IM, Parry-Billings M, Newsholme EA, Fairburn CG and Cowen PJ (1990) Dieting reduces plasma tryptophan and alters brain 5HT function in women. *Psychological Medicine* **20** (4) 785–791.

Bailer UF, Frank GK, Henry SE, Price JC, Meltzer CC, Becker C, Ziolko SK, Mathis CA, Wagner A, Barbarich-Marsteller NC, Putnam K and Kaye WH (2007) Serotonin transporter binding after recovery from eating disorders. *Psychopharmacology (Berl)* **195** (3) 315–324.

Bailer UF, Frank GK, Henry SE, Price JC, Meltzer CC, Weissfeld L, Mathis CA, Drevets WC, Wagner A, Hoge J, Ziolko SK, McConaha CW and Kaye WH (2005) Altered brain serotonin 5-HT1A receptor binding after recovery from anorexia nervosa measured by positron emission tomography and [carbonyl11C]WAY-100635. *Archives of General Psychiatry* **62** (9) 1032–1041.

Becker AE, Grinspoon SK, Klibanski A and Herzog DB (1999) Eating disorders. *The New England Journal of Medicine* **340** (14) 1092–1098.

Brand Miller J, Colagiuri S and Foster-Powell K (1997) The glycemic index is easy and works in practice. *Diabetes Care* **20** (10) 1628–1629.

Bruch H (1985) Four decades of eating disorders. In: DM Garner and PE Garfinkel (Eds) (1997) *Handbook of Treatment For Eating Disorders* (2nd edition). New York: Guilford Press.

Bruinsma K and Taren DL (2000) Dieting, essential fatty acid intake, and depression. *Nutrition Reviews* **58** (4) 98–108.

Colantuoni C, Rada P, McCarthy J, Patten C, Avena NM, Chadeayne A and Hoebel BG (2002) Evidence that intermittent, excessive sugar intake causes endogenous opioid dependence. *Obesity Research* **10** (6) 478–488.

Cowen PJ, Clifford EM, Walsh AE, Williams C and Fairburn CG (1996) Moderate dieting causes 5-HT2C receptor supersensitivity. *Psychological Medicine* **26** (6) 1155–1159.

Curry KR and Jaffe A (1998) *Nutrition Counselling and Communication Skills*. Pennsylvania: WB Saunders Company.

Draper A, Lewis J, Malhotra N and Wheeler E (1993) The energy and nutrient intakes of different types of vegetarian: a case for supplements? *British Journal of Nutrition* **69** (1) 3–19.

Drewnowski A, Krahn DD, Demitrack MA, Nairn K and Gosnell BA (1992) Taste responses and preferences for sweet high-fat foods: evidence for opioid involvement. *Physiology and Behavior* **51** (2) 371–379.

Fairburn CG and Harrison PJ (2003) Eating disorders. *The Lancet* **361** (9355) 407–416.

Fairburn CG and Hill AJ (2005) Eating disorders. In: C Geissler and H Powers (Eds) *Human Nutrition* (11th edition). London: Elsevier, Churchill, Livingstone.

Frost G and Dornhorst A (2000) The relevance of the glycaemic index to our understanding of dietary carbohydrates. *Diabetic Medicine* **17** (5) 336–345.

Garfinkel PE (2002) Classification and diagnosis of eating disorders In: KD Brownell and CG Fairburn (Eds) *Eating Disorders and Obesity: A comprehensive handbook* (2nd edition). New York: Guilford Press.

Garner DM (1997) Psychoeducational principles in treatment. In: DM Garner and PE Garfinkel (Eds) *Handbook of Treatment for Eating Disorders* (2nd edition). New York: Guilford Press.

Gilbody SM, Kirk SF and Hill AJ (1999) Vegetarianism in young women: another means of weight control? *International Journal of Eating Disorders* **26** (1) 87–90.

Golden NH and Meyer W (2004) Nutritional rehabilitation of anorexia nervosa. Goals and dangers. *International Journal of Adolescent Medicine and Health* **16** (2) 131–144.

Harvard Eating Disorders Center (2006–2008) *Who is at Risk?* Available at: www.harriscentermgh.org [accessed 14/07/08].

Herrin M (1999) Balancing the scales. Nutritional counseling for women with eating disorders. *AWHONN Lifelines* **3** (4) 26–34.

Herrin M (2003) *Nutrition Counselling in the Treatment of Eating Disorders*. New York: Brunner Routledge.

Janelle KC and Barr SIJ (1995) Nutrient intakes and eating behavior scores of vegetarian and nonvegetarian women. *Journal of the American Dietetic Association* **95** (2) 180–186.

Johnson WG, Jarrell MP, Chupurdia KM and Williamson DA (1994) Repeated binge/purge cycles in bulimia nervosa: role of glucose and insulin. *International Journal of Eating Disorders* **15** (4) 331–341.

Kaplan AS and Cliska D (1999) The relationship between eating disorders and obesity: psychopathologic and treatment consideration. *Psychiatric Annuals* **29** (4) 197–202.

Kaye W (2007) Neurobiology of anorexia and bulimia nervosa. *Physiology and Behavior* **94** (1) 121–135.

Kaye WH and Weltzin TE (1991) Serotonin activity in anorexia and bulimia nervosa: relationship to the modulation of feeding and mood. *Journal of Clinical Psychiatry* **52** (S12) 41–48.

Keys A, Brozek J, Henschel A, Mickelsen O and Taylor HL (1950) *The Biology of Human Starvation* (2 vols). Minneapolis: University of Minnesota Press.

Logan AC (2003) Neurobehavioral aspects of omega-3 fatty acids: possible mechanisms and therapeutic value in major depression. *Alternative Medicine Review* **8** (4) 410–425.

McFarland B (1995) *Brief Therapy and Eating Disorders.* San Francisco: Jossey-Bass.

Mehler PS (2003) Osteoporosis in anorexia nervosa: prevention and treatment. *International Journal of Eating Disorders* **33** (2) 113–126.

Mercer ME and Holder MD (1997) Food cravings, endogenous opioid peptides, and food intake: a review. *Appetite* **29** (3) 325–352.

Millar HR (1998) New eating disorder service. *Psychiatric Bulletin* **22** 751–754.

Naessén S (2007) *Endocrine and Metabolic Disorders in Bulimic Women and Effects of Antiandrogenic Treatment.* Stockholm: Karolinska Institutet.

National Institute for Clinical Excellence (2004) *Eating Disorders: Core interventions in the treatment and management of anorexia nervosa, bulimia nervosa and related eating disorders.* London: National Institute for Clinical Excellence.

O'Connor TM, O'Halloran DJ and Shanahan F (2000) The stress response and the hypothalamic-pituitary-adrenal axis: from molecule to melancholia. *QJM* **93** (6) 323–333.

Pelchat ML (2002) Of human bondage: food craving, obsession, compulsion, and addiction. *Physiology and Behavior* **76** (3) 347–352.

Pirke KM, Schweiger U, Laessle R, Dickhaut D, Schweiger M and Waechtler M (1986) Dieting influences the menstrual cycle: vegetarian versus non-vegetarian diet. *Fertility and Sterility* **46** (6) 1083–1088.

Ricca V, Mannucci E, Mezani B, di Bernardo M, Zucchi T, Paionni A, Placidi GP, Rotella CM and Faravelli C (2001) Psychopathological and clinical features of outpatients with an eating disorder not otherwise specified. *Eating and Weight Disorders* **6** 157–165.

Rolls BJ, Hetherington M and Burley VJ (1988) The specificity of satiety: the influence of foods of different macronutrient content on the development of satiety. *Physiology and Behavior* **43** (2) 145–153.

Rome ES and Ammerman SJ (2003) Medical complications of eating disorders: an update. *Journal of Adolescent Health* **33** (6) 418–426.

Schebendach J and Nussbaum MP (1992) Nutritional management in adolescents with eating disorders. *Adolescent Medicine: State of the art reviews* **3** (3) 541–558.

Silverman JA (1997) Anorexia nervosa: historical perspective on treatment. In: DM Garner and PE Garfinkel (Eds) (1997) *Handbook of Treatment for Eating Disorders* (2nd edition). New York: Guilford Press.

Sizer FS and Whitney E (2000) *Nutrition: Concepts and controversies* (8th edition). Belmont: Wadsworth.

Sullivan V and Damani S (2000) Vegetarianism and eating disorders: partners in crime? *European Eating Disorders Review* **8** (4) 263–266.

Turner H and Bryant-Waught R (2004) Eating disorder not otherwise specified (EDNOS) profiles of client presenting at a community eating disorder service. *European Eating Disorders Review* **12** (1) 18–26.

Volkow ND, Wang GJ, Fowler JS, Logan J, Jayne M, Franceschi D, Wong C, Gatley SJ, Gifford AN, Ding YS and Pappas N (2002) 'Nonhedonic' food motivation in humans involves dopamine in the dorsal striatum and methylphenidate amplifies this effect. *Synapse* **144** (3) 175–180.

Weltzin TE, Fernstrom MH, Fernstrom JD, Neuberger SK and Kaye WH (1995) Acute tryptophan depletion and increased food intake and irritability in bulimia nervosa. *American Journal of Psychiatry* **152** (11) 1668–1671.

Willard SG, Anding RA and Winstead DK (1983) Nutritional counselling as an adjunct to psychotherapy in bulimia treatment. *Psychosomatics* **24** (6) 545–551.

Winston A, Gowers S, Jackson A, Richardson K, Shenkin A and Williams K (2004) *Guidelines for the Nutritional Management of Anorexia Nervosa*. London: Royal College of Psychiatrists, Eating Disorder Special Interest Group.

Wolfe BE, Metzger ED and Stollar C (1997) The effects of dieting on plasma tryptophan concentration and food intake in healthy women. *Physiological Behaviour* **61** (4) 537–541.

Wurtman RJ and Wurtman JJ (1996) Brain serotonin, carbohydrate-craving, obesity and depression. *Advances in Experimental Medicine and Biology* **398** 35–41.

Chapter 13

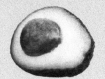

Eat yourself happy – nutritional therapy in practice

CAROLINE STOKES

Nutrition and depression

The occurrence of depression in Western countries is growing at an alarming rate. The number of prescriptions written for antidepressant drugs in England almost tripled from 9.9 million in 1992 to 27.7 million in 2003 (Mental Health Foundation, 2005). In the US the rate of major depression among adults rose from 3.33% to 7.06% between 1991–1992 and 2001–2002 (Compton *et al*, 2006). While depression now affects at least 10% of the population at one point in their lifetime (Gelder *et al*, 1996), it is also commonly seen in young adults and children. This is because the age of onset of the disease is steadily decreasing (Klerman and Weissmann, 1989). Furthermore, there is an increasingly high cost attached to depressive disorders. For example, in England it is estimated that in 2000, the direct and indirect cost for the treatment of depressive disorders amounted to approximately £9 billion (Thomas and Morris, 2003). These numbers will rise quickly, as depression is predicted to be the number two disabling disease on a global scale after cardiovascular disease by the year 2020 (Murray and Lopez, 1997).

The usual treatment for depression entails drug therapy and psychotherapy. Because of the high cost, possible side effects of drugs, potential lack of response to the treatment and excessively long waiting lists for treatment within the public healthcare system, alternative and supplementary treatment approaches can be of significant importance for the prevention and treatment of depression. The human brain has significant nutrient and energy needs, and this makes it surprising that the role of nutrition on mental health status is often overlooked. For example, the 2003 World Health Organization report on *Diet, Nutrition and the Prevention of Chronic Diseases* (2003) does not acknowledge mental health as a nutrition-related disease.

There is significant evidence linking reduced levels of certain nutrients to the occurrence and intensity of mental health disorders among the population. For example, ecological studies have shown international variations in rates of depression to correlate with fish consumption in the national diet (Peet, 2004) and in populations with low fish consumption individuals are reported to have an increased risk of depression (Tanskanen *et al*, 2001). Another study investigated fish intake in 23 countries and found lower incidence of postpartum depression among those countries with higher fish consumption (Hibbeln, 2002). Furthermore, population-based observational studies report an inverse relationship between omega-3 fatty acid, folate, selenium and zinc blood concentrations and levels of depressive symptoms. As a result, there is the potential to use nutritional supplementation to prevent mental health problems.

There is clinical trial evidence showing that nutritional approaches can be of significant benefit in the management of depression. The evidence largely concentrates on nutrient-based interventions through the use of nutritional supplements, however, data on food-based interventions is limited. For example, clinical trials with supplementation of omega-3 fatty acids, folic acid and tryptophan are reported as being beneficial in the treatment of depression as an adjunct to antidepressant medication. Some clinical trials support a positive influence of zinc, chromium and vitamins B12 and B6 and there is also suggestive evidence that selenium may be beneficial for depression. These nutrients are discussed in more detail in the following section.

How can you eat yourself happy?

The connection between food and depressive disorders has been clearly established in epidemiological studies. The important question is, of course, which are the nutrients that affect depression and how much has to be consumed to help reduce the symptoms of the disease? Much of the research into the biochemical causes of depression focuses on neurotransmitters, such as serotonin. As a result, nutrients that affect neurotransmitter levels are believed to be important for treating depression.

The introduction to this chapter mentions several long-term epidemiological studies that demonstrate significant correlations between certain active nutrients and their role in reducing the extent of depressive symptoms. The more practical information given in this section is derived from clinical trials, where effects are observed over a much shorter period of time (usually months). This is important, as the short-term efficacy of certain nutrients allows them to be used for immediate treatment of depressive disorders.

There are a number of nutrients for which clear clinical evidence is available, showing their efficacy in reducing symptoms of depression. The two most significant are omega-3 fatty acids and folic acid. Additionally, there is good supporting data for tryptophan, zinc and vitamin B12. Finally, vitamin B6, chromium and selenium have also shown preliminary success in some studies but require more clinical research to fully prove their positive roles. In the following sections some of the clinical evidence for these nutrients is discussed along with essential information on the food sources for obtaining them.

Omega-3 fatty acids

The most convincing scientific evidence for the positive effects of nutrition on mental health disorders comes from studies utilising polyunsaturated fatty acids (PUFA) such as omega-3 fatty acids. It has been shown that depression is more common in people with low serum and red blood cell concentrations of omega-3 fatty acids (Peet *et al*, 1998). Also, people with depression suffer from reduced serotonin uptake (Mellerup and Plenge, 1988). Thus, low blood concentrations of omega-3 fatty acids may contribute to depression by reducing membrane fluidity and negatively impacting the transport of serotonin into the endothelial cells (Block and Edwards, 1987).

Several well-controlled trials have found supplementation with eicosapentaenoic acid (EPA), a long chain PUFA, to result in improvements in symptoms of depression (Peet and Horrobin, 2002; Frangou *et al*, 2006). Most of these studies are based on adults, but a similar study in children also showed the same results (Nemets *et al*, 2006). These interventions typically supplemented the subjects with ~1 g of ethyl-EPA per day; greater doses did not produce any significant improvements in depressive symptoms compared with the placebo. An overview of omega-3 fatty acids in the treatment of depression has recently been published (Peet and Stokes, 2005). Omega-3 fatty acids can be obtained from oily fish such as salmon, mackerel, sardines, herring and fresh tuna.

The UK government at present recommends that we consume two portions of fish per week, of which one should be an oily fish. Further, a maximum level of consumption for oily fish is set at four oily fish meals per week (about 140 grams per portion) for the general population. This excludes pregnant and lactating women and girls or women who might have a child one day. For this group, the maximum recommendation is set at two oily fish meals per week (SACN/COT, 2004). Another good source for omega-3 fatty acids, particularly for vegetarians, are flaxseeds or flaxseed oil (also known as linseeds/linseed oil), which contain the precursor fatty acid, α-linolenic acid (ALA). ALA is converted to EPA in the body after ingestion, however the rate of conversion can vary among individuals and may also be affected by external factors.

Omega-3 fatty acids have a multitude of other health benefits: they have been shown to reduce the risk of coronary heart disease, stroke and conditions such as rheumatic arthritis as well as reduce triglyceride levels in the blood. However, there is a need for further research focusing on food sources of omega-3 fatty acids in the treatment of depression, since the doses used for treatment may be difficult to obtain from *diet* alone.

Folate (folic acid)

Folate (or folic acid) is a B vitamin. Prior to discussing the evidence base, however, one important distinction needs to be made between folate and folic acid. Folate is the natural form of this vitamin, which is naturally present in some foods. Folic acid, on the other hand, is the man-made form of this vitamin, which is used in nutritional supplements or added in foods, such as bread and breakfast cereals, in order to fortify them with folic acid. Throughout this chapter, the relevant terminology will be used depending on which form of the vitamin is being discussed.

Depression has also been associated with lower concentrations of serum and red cell folate, typically in those individuals with folate values at the lower end of the dietary reference value (Morris *et al*, 2003). Wesson *et al* (1994) reported an inverse relationship between folate blood levels and severity of depression. Furthermore, Papakostas *et al* (2004) found low folate concentrations to be a marker for a poor response to antidepressant treatment in a study of 14 patients with major depression.

Several controlled trials supplementing folic acid to people with depression showed significant improvements in response to the antidepressant medication (Coppen and Bailey, 2000; Abou-Saleh and Coppen, 2006). The dosages used in the above studies were very similar to current intake values, therefore, dietary intake from the daily consumption of foods containing folate, such as green leafy vegetables, citrus fruits and foods containing folic acid such as fortified breads and breakfast cereals (***Table 1***) should provide the necessary levels of folic acid.

Folate is also required for the formation of healthy red blood cells and it reduces the risk of birth defects such as spina bifida in unborn babies.

Tryptophan

There is good evidence for the efficacy of tryptophan for treating depression as an adjunct to antidepressant medication in controlled trials (Levitan *et al*, 2000). Tryptophan is an amino acid found in protein foods, such as meat and dairy products, and is also available on prescription in the UK. Tryptophan is a biochemical precursor for serotonin, hence its important role in mental health disorders linked to low serotonin levels in the brain. Fortunately, it is easily possible to obtain sufficient quantities of tryptophan from dietary sources (***Table 1***).

The evidence for the usefulness of other nutrients is less complete, however, it is elaborated on below. Refer to ***Table 1*** for the corresponding food sources.

Zinc

A study comparing zinc concentrations in serum found them to be significantly lower in patients with major depression than in healthy controls (McLoughlin and Hodge, 1990; Maes *et al*, 1994). Maes *et al* (1994) also reported a negative correlation between the severity of depression and serum zinc concentrations, corroborated by findings of low plasma concentrations of zinc in people with depression.

A controlled trial supplementing zinc to adults with depression found it to augment their antidepressant therapy (Nowak *et al*, 2005). The authors used a relatively high dosage of 25 mg of zinc per day, which could, nevertheless, be readily obtained from food sources such as wholemeal bread, cereal products, meat, fish, dairy products and pumpkin seeds (***Table 1***).

Zinc also helps to maintain a healthy immune system and is needed for wound healing.

TABLE 1: SUMMARY OF MAIN FOOD SOURCES FOR IMPORTANT NUTRIENTS IN DEPRESSION

Nutrient	Food sources
Omega-3 fatty acids	Oily fish (mackerel, salmon, sardines, herrings, fresh tuna), flaxseeds/oil, walnuts
Folic acid	Green leafy vegetables (broccoli, spinach), citrus fruits, fortified breads and breakfast cereals
Tryptophan	Meat, poultry, fish, eggs, low-fat dairy products (milk, yoghurt, cheese), bananas
Zinc	Meat, shellfish, low-fat dairy foods (milk, cheese), bread, and cereal products such as wheatgerm, pumpkin seeds
Chromium	Meat, wholegrains such as wholemeal bread and whole oats, lentils, spices
Selenium	Brazil nuts, bread, fish, meat, eggs
Vitamin B6	Pork, chicken, turkey, cod, bread, whole cereals (oatmeal, rice), eggs, vegetables, peanuts, milk, potatoes
Vitamin B12	Meat, salmon, cod, milk, cheese, eggs, yeast extract, some fortified breakfast cereals

Vitamin B12

Low blood concentrations of vitamin B12 have been reported in depressed patients compared with non-depressed patients (Penninx *et al*, 2000; Bjelland *et al*, 2003). Tiemeier *et al* (2002) also found that subjects with low blood vitamin B12 concentrations were 70% more likely to suffer from severe depression compared with subjects with normal to high concentrations. A recent study suggests that high vitamin B12 status may be associated with better treatment outcome (Coppen and Bolander-Gouaille, 2005).

Vitamin B12 is also needed to keep the nervous system healthy and helps to process folic acid. It can be obtained from a variety of food sources, such as meat, salmon, cod, milk, cheese, eggs, yeast extract and some fortified breakfast cereals.

Vitamin B6, chromium and selenium

A systematic review by Williams *et al* (2005), including five controlled trials and one intervention study, concluded that there is consistent evidence in support of vitamin B6 supplementation for the treatment of depression in pre-menopausal women but not for depression in general. Therefore, more research is needed to confirm these preliminary findings. Similar preliminary evidence was found for chromium. A controlled trial supplementing 600 mcg of chromium per day was shown to be effective in people with major depression (Davidson *et al*, 2003). For selenium, a study in healthy volunteers indicates that low selenium status is associated with depressed mood (Rayman, 2002). Controlled trials have reported improved mood scores in subjects supplemented with 100–150 mcg of selenium compared with those receiving a placebo (Bodnar and Wisner, 2005). Food sources for vitamin B6, chromium and selenium are summarised in **Table 1** (previous page).

Synergistic influences

Some research has shown that health-promoting behaviours, such as eating breakfast and having regular meals, especially home-cooked family meals, are also protective against depression as, among other benefits, they may encourage following a healthy diet and increase the likelihood of obtaining the necessary nutrients (Lombard, 2000; Fulkerson *et al*, 2004). Furthermore, significant evidence demonstrates the beneficial role of physical activity in the treatment of depression (Manger and Motta, 2005). In some cases physical activity can be as effective as cognitive behavioural therapy, as outlined in two recent review articles (Barbour *et al*, 2007; Miles, 2007). Finally, the present author's previous research within the NHS involved setting up a 'Mood and Lifestyle Clinic' as a pilot project, offering nutritional approaches and physical activity to people suffering from depression (Stokes, 2006). The project enabled clients to make appropriate adjustments to their diets and to include more physical activity into their daily lives (a supplementary DVD presents additional data and advice: Peet and Stokes, 2005).

Conclusions

There is a curious lack of knowledge and awareness of the relationship between nutrition and depression. This is somewhat surprising, as the beneficial effects of certain nutrients on the mental health state of people suffering from depressive disorders have clearly been demonstrated in clinical studies (Bodnar and Wisner, 2005; Bamber *et al*, 2007). Obviously, large-scale, well-controlled trials are required to provide more quantitative and conclusive evidence, to fully explore the intrinsic links between nutrition and its role in the treatment of depression. To date, the evidence has tended to focus on nutrient-based studies, which entail the use of supplements. However, there is clearly a need for further research in the form of food-based studies, focusing on food sources of the nutrients mentioned above, particularly because in some cases, such as omega-3 fatty acids, doses used for the nutritional therapy may be difficult to obtain from *diet* alone. There is sufficient data available, however, to support the provision of practical nutritional therapies for depression at this point.

The nutrients discussed in this chapter have all been linked to alleviating depressed moods and thus can be recommended for the adjunctive treatment of depressive disorders. Importantly, these essential components are part of any normal, healthy diet, and they can be obtained from a variety of food sources. There is no harm in trying these approaches, as long as well-trained nutritionists give proper advice and differentiate between dosages and the amounts one would obtain from normal food sources, especially if nutritional supplements are taken. Interestingly, many people suffering from depression use dietary manipulation as a form of self-help. For example, eating more fish, fruit and vegetables and reducing sugar and saturated fat intake, is an approach favoured by service users as shown by the success from the MIND Food and Mood project (Geary, 2001). Ideally, nutritional approaches should be incorporated into integrated care pathways, so that a standard care package that includes dietary advice can be routinely offered to those wishing to treat their depressive symptoms. This is the advice that has recently been supported by the Associate Parliamentary Food and Health Forum in their 2008 report on the links between diet and behaviour.

In summary, this chapter has naturally focused on those nutrients for which some experimental evidence is available to support their use in treatment protocols. There are certainly many other potential nutrients, such as antioxidants, for which little clinical evidence for their positive role in depression has yet been shown. Furthermore, most of the clinical evidence in nutritional correlation studies of food and mental health is derived from very small clinical trials. It is important, in the future, to conduct long-term and large-scale clinical studies to supplement the data from epidemiological studies.

The author hopes that the convincing information available to date for some nutrients will encourage nutritional scientists to conduct further research in this largely unexplored area of science and that funding bodies will provide the necessary support for the research. Ultimately, regulatory agencies and the government should provide practical advice to the public on the beneficial effects of nutritional treatment for depression once more research has conclusively proven the clinical observations seen to date.

References

Abou-Saleh MT and Coppen A (2006) Folic acid and the treatment of depression. *Journal of Psychosomatic Research* **61** (3) 285–287.

Associate Parliamentary Food and Health Forum (2008) *The Links between Diet and Behaviour: The influence of nutrition on mental health.* London: Associate Parliamentary Food and Health Forum.

Bamber DJ, Stokes CS and Stephen AM (2007) The role of diet in the prevention and management of adolescent depression. *Nutrition Bulletin* **31** (S1) 90–99.

Barbour KA, Edenfield TM and Blumenthal JA (2007) Exercise as a treatment for depression and other psychiatric disorders: a review. *Journal of Cardiopulmonary Rehabilitation and Prevention* **27** (6) 359–367.

Bjelland I, Tell GS, Vollset SE, Refsum H and Ueland PM (2003) Folate, vitamin B12, homocysteine, and the MTHFR 677C->T polymorphism in anxiety and depression: the Hordaland Homocysteine study. *Archives of General Psychiatry* **60** (6) 618–626.

Block ER and Edwards D (1987) Effect of plasma membrane fluidity on serotonin transport by endothelial cells. *American Journal of Physiology* **253** (5) C672–C678.

Bodnar LM and Wisner KL (2005) Nutrition and depression: implications for improving mental health among childbearing-aged women. *Biological Psychiatry* **58** (9) 679–685.

Compton WM, Conway KP, Stinson FS and Grant BF (2006) Changes in the prevalence of major depression comorbid substance use disorders in the United States between 1991–1992 and 2001–2002. *American Journal of Psychiatry* **163** (12) 2141–2147.

Coppen A and Bailey J (2000) Enhancement of the antidepressant action of fluoxetine by folic acid: a randomised, placebo controlled trial. *Journal of Affective Disorders* **60** (2) 121–130.

Coppen A and Bolander-Gouaille C (2005) Treatment of depression: time to consider folic acid and vitamin B12. *Journal of Psychopharmacology* **19** (1) 59–65.

Davidson JR, Abraham K, Connor KM and McLeod M (2003) Effectiveness of chromium in atypical depression: a placebo-controlled trial. *Biological Psychiatry* **53** (3) 261–264.

Frangou S, Lewis M and McCrone P (2006) Efficacy of ethyl-eicosapentaenoic acid in bipolar depression: randomised double-blind placebo-controlled study. *British Journal of Psychiatry* **188** (1) 46–50.

Fulkerson JA, Sherwood NE, Perry CL, Neumark-Sztainer D and Story M (2004) Depressive symptoms and adolescent eating and health behaviours: a multifaceted view in a population-based sample. *Preventive Medicine* **38** (6) 865–875.

Geary A (2001) *The Food and Mood Handbook.* London: Thorson's Publishers.

Gelder M, Gath D, Mayou R and Cowen P (1996) *Oxford Textbook of Psychiatry.* Oxford: Oxford University Press.

Hibbeln JR (2002) Seafood consumption, the DHA content of mothers' milk, and prevalence rates of postpartum depression: a cross-national, ecological analysis. *Journal of Affective Disorders* **69** (1) 15–29.

Klerman GL and Weissmann MM (1989) Increasing rates of depression. *JAMA* **261** (15) 2229–2235.

Levitan RD, Shen JH, Jindal R, Driver HS, Kennedy HS and Shapiro CM (2000) Preliminary randomized double-blind placebo-controlled trial of tryptophan combined with fluoxetine to treat major depressive disorder: antidepressant and hypnotic effects. *Journal of Psychiatry and Neuroscience* **25** (4) 337–346.

Lombard CB (2000) What is the role of food in preventing depression and improving mood performance and cognitive function? *Medical Journal of Australia* **173** S104-105.

Maes M, d'Haese PC, Scharpe S, d'Hondt P, Cosyns P and de Broe ME (1994) Hypozincemia in depression. *Journal of Affective Disorders* **31** (2) 135–140.

Manger TA and Motta RW (2005) The impact of an exercise program on posttraumatic stress disorder, anxiety and depression. *International Journal of Emergency Mental Health* **7** (1) 49–57.

McLoughlin IJ and Hodge JS (1990) Zinc in depressive disorder. *Acta Psychiatrica Scandinavica* **82** (6) 451–453.

Mellerup ET and Plenge P (1988) Imipramine binding in depression and other psychiatric conditions. *Acta Psychiatrica Scandinavica* **345** S61–S68.

Mental Health Foundation (2005) *Up and Running. Exercise therapy and the treatment of mild or moderate depression in primary care.* London: Mental Health Foundation.

Miles L (2007) Physical activity and health. *Nutrition Bulletin* **32** (4) 314–363.

Morris MS, Fava M, Jacques PF, Selhub J and Rosenberg IH (2003) Depression and folate status in the US population. *Psychotherapy and Psychosomatics* **72** (2) 80–87.

Murray CJ and Lopez AD (1997) Alternative projections of mortality and disability by cause 1990–2020: global burden of disease study. *The Lancet* **349** (9064) 1498–1504.

Nemets H, Nemets V, Apter A, Brachta Z and Belmaker RH (2006) Omega-3 treatment of childhood depression: a controlled, double-blind study. *American Journal of Psychiatry* **163** (6) 1098–1100.

Nowak G, Szewczyk B and Pilc A (2005) Zinc and depression. An update. *Pharmacological Reports* **57** (6) 713–718.

Papakostas GI, Petersen T, Mischoulon D, Ryan JL, Nierenberg AA, Bottiglieri T, Rosenbaum JF, Alpert JE and Fava M (2004) Serum folate, vitamin B12, and homocysteine in major depressive disorder. Part 1: predictors of clinical response in fluoxetine-resistant depression. *Journal of Clinical Psychiatry* **65** (8) 1090–1095.

Peet M (2004) International variations in the outcome of schizophrenia and the prevalence of depression in relation to national dietary practices: an ecological analysis. *British Journal of Psychiatry* **184** (5) 404–408.

Peet M and Horrobin DF (2002) A dose-ranging study of the effects of ethyl-eicosapentaenoate in patients with ongoing depression despite apparently adequate treatment with standard drugs. *Archives of General Psychiatry* **59** (10) 913–919.

Peet M and Stokes C (2005) *Eat Yourself Happy.* DVD available from: www.nhs-ennovations.com/index.php?cPath=25 [accessed 22/05/08].

Peet M and Stokes C (2005) Omega-3 fatty acids in the treatment of psychiatric disorders. *Drugs* **65** (8) 1051–1059.

Peet M, Murphy B, Shay J and Horrobin D (1998) Depletion of omega-3 fatty acid levels in red blood cells membranes of depressive patients. *Biological Psychiatry* **43** (5) 315–319.

Penninx B, Guralnik JM, Ferrucci L, Fried LP, Allen RH and Stabler SP (2000) Vitamin B12 deficiency and depression in physically disabled older women: epidemiologic evidence from the women's health and aging study. *American Journal of Psychiatry* **157** (5) 715–721.

Rayman MP (2002) The importance of selenium to human health. *The Lancet* **356** (2000) 233–241.

SACN/COT (Scientific Advisory Committee on Nutrition/Committee of Toxicity) (2004) *Advice on Fish Consumption: Benefits and risks.* The Stationery Office: Norwich.

Stokes C (2006) A nutritional approach to the treatment of depression: the mood and lifestyle clinic. *The Nutrition Practitioner* **7** 53–55.

Tanskanen A, Hibbeln JR, Tuomilehto J, Tuomilehto J, Uutela A, Haukkala A, Viinamäki H, Lehtonen J and Vartiainen E (2001) Fish consumption and depressive symptoms in the general population in Finland. *Psychiatric Services* **52** (4) 529–531.

Thomas CM and Morris S (2003) Cost of depression among adults in England. *The British Journal of Psychiatry* **183** (6) 514–519.

Tiemeier H, van Tuijl HR, Hofman A, Meijer J, Kiliaan AJ and Breteler MMB (2002) Vitamin B12, folate, and homocysteine in depression: the Rotterdam study. *American Journal of Psychiatry* **159** (12) 2099–2101.

Wesson VA, Levitt AJ and Joffe RT (1994) Change in folate status with antidepressant treatment. *Psychiatry Research* **53** (3) 313–322.

Williams AL, Cotter A, Sabina A, Girard C, Goodman J and Katz DL (2005) The role for vitamin B6 as treatment for depression: a systematic review. *Family Practice* **22** (5) 532–537.

World Health Organization (2003) *Diet, Nutrition and the Prevention of Chronic Diseases.* World Health Organization Technical Report Series 916. Geneva: Joint World Health Organization/Food and Agriculture Organization Expert Consultation.

Editor's summary
Twenty strategies to support a healthy mind

MARTINA WATTS

1. Rehydrate regularly throughout the day – preferably with just water (add a slice of lemon or lime if preferred).

2. Eat regular meals and try to have breakfast, even if it's just fruit. Support digestion by eating slowly and chewing food well.

3. Eat a healthy diet. This means a diet with a high nutrient density, containing vitamins, minerals, antioxidants, phytonutrients, amino acids and polyunsaturated fatty acids. *Chapter 1* provides guidelines concerning our genetic 'compatibility' with certain foods.

4. Look for a variety of fresh, colourful, local and seasonal produce and try to eat five to eight portions per day (raw, steamed or stir-fried). *Chapter 2* shows how to prevent mineral losses.

5. Buy whole basic ingredients of high quality, and clean, assemble, cook and bake them at home. Avoid refined grains and eat a variety of wholegrain products. Wholegrains consist of the entire grain seed of a plant, including the bran, germ and endosperm. Wheat, barley, rye and triticale contain gluten. Oats do not contain gluten, but may be contaminated with gluten. Quinoa, amaranth, buckwheat groats, corn, millet, brown or wild rice, sorghum and teff are gluten-free.

6. Eat quality protein every day (meat, fish, eggs, dairy from reputable sources). If vegetarian, combine wholegrains with beans and pulses.

7. Eat two to four portions of fish per week (pregnant and lactating women or women trying to conceive should have a maximum of two portions and consider supplementing with fish oil, not cod liver oil, from a reputable source). For mood disorders, a fish-oil supplement containing one gram of EPA and DHA per day may be helpful (ensure it is free of harmful residues by buying from a reputable supplier). *Chapter 6* provides detailed information on the importance of omega-3 fish oils.

8. Avoid common blood sugar disrupters: sugar and other forms of concentrated sweetness (including artificial sweeteners), caffeine, nicotine, alcohol, stress. *Chapter 11* explains how to balance blood sugar levels.

9. Avoid added salt (sodium chloride) or salty convenience foods.

10. Eat the right fats. The oils in fish, nuts, seeds, avocados and olives are highly beneficial. Avoid hydrogenated and deep-fried fats.

11. Read labels and look for items that do not have a long list of additives (check drinks, toothpaste and medicines as well). **Chapter 3** provides a list of additives and alternatives.

12. If you suspect an allergy to mercury, consider having mercury amalgams removed by an informed dentist. **Chapter 4** reveals the difference between mercury toxicity and allergy.

13. Identify any suspected food intolerances with the help of an experienced nutrition practitioner. **Chapter 10** describes testing procedures most likely to be reliable.

14. Improve intestinal bacterial flora by taking probiotics from a reputable source, including lactic acid and bifido bacteria. If intestinal pathogens are suspected, they should be tested for and removed. **Chapter 5** and **Chapter 7** explain how the bacterial flora in your gut can affect your mental health.

15. Be aware that de-junking your diet can make you feel worse before you feel better, due to withdrawal symptoms or poor liver detoxification. Anyone with mood disorders should be made fully aware that they may suddenly feel more depressed or anxious for a short period of time following dietary changes, particularly after avoiding sugar, refined carbohydrates, caffeine, dairy or gluten. Make any changes to your diet slowly and seek professional advice.

16. Do not stop taking any medication without prior consultation with your doctor.

17. People with mood disorders may have individual nutrient requirements (see **Chapter 8**, **Chapter 9** and **Chapter 13**). Do not self-medicate, consult a qualified nutrition practitioner. To find one in your area consult your GP or visit www.bant.org.uk.

18. Eating disorders are complex mental health conditions and care must include psychological treatments and regular medical monitoring. **Chapter 12** outlines different types of eating disorders.

19. Ensure adequate sleep and daily exercise.

20. Increase fresh air and sunlight.

Glossary

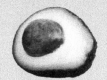

Acetylcholine
A neurotransmitter synthesised in the human body from dietary choline, a natural substance found in lecithin, and a two-carbon molecule called acetyl.

Alpha-ketoglutaric acid
An organic acid that is important for the proper metabolism of all essential amino acids and the transfer of cellular energy.

Alpha-linolenic acid (ALA)
An essential fatty acid found in flaxseed and walnuts.

Alpha lipoic acid
A water- and fat-soluble substance found in the body and certain foods, serves as a potent antioxidant.

Amino acid
An organic acid and building unit from which proteins are formed.

Amphetamine
A drug with a stimulant effect on the central nervous system that can be both physically and psychologically addictive when abused (also known as 'speed').

Anaemia
A condition where someone has an abnormally low amount of red blood cells, or less than the normal quantity of haemoglobin, in the blood.

Anaphylaxis
A sudden, severe and life-threatening allergic reaction to an allergen.

Anhedonia
The inability to gain pleasure from normally pleasurable experiences.

Anorexia nervosa
An eating disorder characterised by markedly reduced appetite or total aversion to food.

Antibody
A protein (immunoglobulin) produced by lymphocytes (white blood cells) in response to a foreign substance called an antigen.

Antigen

A foreign substance that induces the production of antibodies by the immune system.

Antioxidant

Any substance that reduces oxidative damage such as that caused by free radicals.

Apo-lipoprotein E (ApoE)

A type of protein connected to a fat and associated with several cardiovascular disorders.

Arachidonic acid (AA)

A polyunsaturated fatty acid present in the membrane phospholipids of body cells, and abundant in the brain.

Asperger's syndrome

One of the autistic spectrum disorders that cause communication problems and social impairment. To people with these disorders the world can appear chaotic with no clear boundaries, order or meaning.

Asthma

A lung disease that causes wheezing, coughing and tightness of the chest, making it difficult to breathe.

Atopic

An inherited tendency to develop an allergy.

Attention deficit disorder (ADD)

Development disorder that impairs one's ability to sustain focus.

Attention deficit hyperactivity disorder (ADHD)

The most common childhood-onset behavioural disorder. The core symptoms include an inability to sustain attention and concentration, and developmentally inappropriate levels of activity, distractibility and impulsivity.

Autism

A spectrum of neuropsychiatric disorders characterised by deficits in social interaction and communication, and unusual and repetitive behaviour. The degree of autism varies from mild to severe in different people.

Bifidobacteria

A form of 'friendly' bacteria that resides in the lower part of the digestive system.

Binge eating disorder

An eating disorder characterised by periods of extreme over-eating.

Bio-dynamically grown foods

Bio-dynamic agriculture is an advanced organic farming system that places emphasis on food quality and soil health.

Biotin

A water-soluble B-complex vitamin.

Bipolar disorder

A mood disorder, sometimes called manic-depression, which characteristically involves cycles of depression and elation or mania.

Blackmore's mineral celloid therapy

A unique drugless therapy developed in Australia by Maurice Blackmore.

Boron

An important mineral for healthy bones, especially for the metabolism of calcium, magnesium, and phosphorus.

Brain-derived neurotrophic factor (BDNF)

A protein that supports the survival of existing neurons and encourages the growth and differentiation of new neurons.

Bulimia nervosa

An eating disorder characterised by episodes of secretive excessive binge-eating followed by self-induced vomiting, abuse of laxatives and diuretics, or excessive exercise.

Casein

The main protein found in milk and other dairy products.

Casomorphine

A particular type of protein fragment with opioid effects derived from incomplete digestion of casein.

Cat's claw

A herb that grows in rainforest and jungle areas in South America and Asia and has been used for centuries to prevent and treat disease.

Chlorella

Freshwater single-cell green algae, popular as a dietary supplement.

Chromium

A trace element found widely in the environment and believed to influence how insulin behaves in the body.

Chronic fatigue syndrome (CFS)

A debilitating and complex disorder characterised by profound fatigue as well as other physical symptoms for six months or longer.

Cortisol

The primary stress hormone.

Cytokines

Small proteins released from white blood cells and other cells, that act as chemical signals between cells.

Delta-6 desaturase

Enzyme that converts linoleic acid to gamma linolenic acid (GLA).

Digestive enzymes

Enzymes in the digestive tract that break down complex substances into simpler ones so they can be absorbed. Available in supplement form.

Dihomogamma-linolenic acid (DGLA)

A highly unsaturated fatty acid from the omega-6 family.

Dimercaptosuccinic acid (DMSA)

A Food and Drug Administration (FDA)-approved sulphur compound used as treatment for heavy metal toxicity.

Docosahexaenoic acid (DHA)

Long-chain polyunsaturated fatty acid – a vital component of the phospholipids of human cellular membranes, especially those in the brain and retina. It is necessary for optimal development.

Dopamine

A major neurotransmitter present in regions of the brain that regulate movement, emotion, motivation and the feeling of pleasure.

Dyslexia

A specific reading disability due to a defect in the brain's processing of graphic symbols.

Dyspraxia

A motor learning disability that affects movement and co-ordination.

Eczema

An itchy, inflammatory skin condition associated with allergy.

Eicosanoids

Signalling molecules derived from omega-3 or omega-6 fats.

Eicosapentaenoic acid (EPA)
A long-chain omega-3 fatty acid found primarily in fish and shellfish.

Essential fatty acid (EFA)
Unsaturated fatty acid essential to human health; it cannot be manufactured in the body.

Feingold diet
A diet intended to treat hyperactive children, which excludes colourings, flavourings, and naturally occurring aspirin-like compounds (salicylates).

Fibromyalgia
A chronic condition causing pain, stiffness and tenderness of the muscles, tendons and joints.

Flavonoids
Water-soluble plant pigments beneficial to human health.

Folate (Folic acid)
One of the B vitamins and a key factor in the synthesis of DNA and RNA.

Glutathione
A major cellular antioxidant needed for immune function and the production of energy.

Gluten
A protein found in wheat, barley or rye. Oats do not have gluten *in* them, but can have gluten *on* them, due to contamination in processing plants, and can therefore trigger a gluten allergy.

Gluteomorphins
Peptides with opioid acitivity due to incomplete digestion of gluten.

Glycaemic index (GI)
Indicator of the ability of different types of foods that contain carbohydrate to raise blood glucose levels within two hours. Carbohydrate-containing foods that break down most quickly during digestion have the highest glycaemic index.

Hallucinogen
A drug, such as LSD, that causes profound distortions in a person's perceptions of reality.

Highly unsaturated fatty acids (HUFAs)
Special kinds of polyunsaturated fats (omega-3 and omega-6) crucial to brain development and function.

Histamine

A naturally occurring substance that is released by the immune system after being exposed to an allergen; also acts as a neurotransmitter.

Hypothalamic-pituitary-adrenal axis (HPA)

A feedback loop that includes the hypothalamus, the pituitary and the adrenal glands.

Hypothalamus

The area of the brain that controls body temperature, hunger and thirst.

Immunoglobulin (Ig)

A glycoprotein that functions as an antibody. There are five classes with different structures (IgA, IgD, IgE, IgG, IgM).

In vitro

Testing outside the body (opposite of in vivo – in the body).

Indole

An organic compound found in the amino acid tryptophan, alkaloids and pigments.

Indoleamine 2, 3-dioxygenase (IDO)

A special enzyme produced in response to stress to help manage immune chemicals and to control the metabolism of tryptophan – an important amino acid in the production of the mood-enhancing neurotransmitter serotonin.

Ion channels

These allow the movement of ions across cell membranes; present in the membranes that surround all biological cells.

Kamut

A high protein wheat variety and an ancient relative of modern durum wheat.

Kefir

A cultured milk drink popular in the Middle East and Eastern Europe, consisting of a complex mixture of lactic acid bacteria and friendly yeasts.

Kelp

A type of marine algae or seaweed.

Kryptopyrroles

Chemicals produced by the body as a by-product of making haemoglobin. Some people suffer from elevated levels of kryptopyrroles, which block receptor sites of vitamin B6 and zinc leading to serious deficiencies of these nutrients.

Kynurenines
Endogenous metabolites of tryptophan metabolism, which may be neurotoxic and cause depressive behaviour and/or neurodegenerative disease.

Lactobacilli
Bacteria found mainly in the mouth, intestinal tract and vagina. Lactobacilli also live in fermenting products, such as live yoghurt.

Leukotrienes
Hormone-like chemicals derived from fatty acids, which contribute to inflammation and allergy.

Limbic system
A network of structures in the brain involved in memory and emotions.

Linoleic acid (LA)
A polyunsaturated fatty acid of the omega-6 family abundant in many vegetable oils.

Macronutrients
Carbohydrate, protein and fat.

Macular degeneration
A disease that progressively destroys the central portion of the retina and may cause blindness.

Memory lymphocyte
A type of white blood cell important in the secondary immune response.

Micronutrients
Needed for life, in small quantities, such as vitamins, minerals, trace elements.

Mitochondria
Cellular structures responsible for energy production.

Molybdenum
A trace element found in a wide variety of foods including nuts, vegetables, and cereals such as oats.

Monounsaturated fatty acids
Fatty acids whose carbon chains have one double bond. Foods high in monounsaturated fats include canola and olive oil.

Myelin basic protein (MBP)
A protein believed to be important in the process of myelination of nerves in the central nervous system (CNS).

N-acetylcysteine (NAC)
Antioxidant agent derived from the amino acid cysteine.

Neuron-axon filament protein (NAFP)
A protein essential for building axons, the branches of nerve cells that carry messages to the next nerve cell.

Neurotransmitter
A messenger of neurological information from one cell to another.

Niacin
One of the B-complex vitamins (also known as vitamin B3, nicotinic acid, nicotinamide, niacinamide).

Noradrenaline (norepinephrine)
Catecholamine neurotransmitter, used by the sympathetic nervous system and in the brain.

NPK fertilisers
NPK represents the key constituent chemical elements nitrogen (N), phosphorus (P) and potassium (K) used in plant fertilisers. Environmentalists and supporters of the organic movement regard these as harmful to health and the environment.

NSAIDs
Non-steroidal anti-inflammatory drugs. They can damage the lining of the stomach and cause bleeding if taken in higher doses over a long period of time, and are also linked to other side effects.

Nuclear factor kappa B
Acts as a cellular specialist in the production of inflammation in the face of infection and certain stressors. It is a sophisticated amplifier of over 400 genes dedicated to increasing inflammation to defend us, which if not controlled can lead to inflammation-based illnesses.

Oedema
Swelling due to the retention of fluids in the tissues.

Omega-3
A class of essential fatty acids found primarily in fish oils, especially from salmon and other cold-water fish. EPA (eicosapentaenoic acid) and DHA (docosahexaenoic acid) are the two principal omega-3 fatty acids.

Omega-6
A class of essential fatty acids found in seeds and nuts, and the oils extracted from them. GLA (Gamma-linolenic acid) is a principle omega-6 fatty acid found primarily in hemp, borage and evening primrose oil.

Omega-9
Monounsaturated fatty acids found in olive oil and avocados. Unlike essential fatty acids, they can be manufactured by the body.

Opioid peptides
Short sequences of amino acids that mimic the effect of opiates in the brain.

Oral allergy syndrome (OAS)
An allergic reaction in hay fever sufferers contained to the mouth and throat, resulting from direct contact with certain fruits, nuts, and vegetables. It is not usually life-threatening (unlike anaphylaxis).

Organelle
Refers to any structure which occurs in a cell and that has a specialised function.

Oxidative stress
Increased oxidant production in cells characterised by the release of free radicals and resulting in cellular degeneration.

Palladium
A silver white metallic element belonging to the platinum group.

Pantothenic acid
Vitamin B5.

Phosphorus
An essential element in the diet and a major component of bone, but also found in blood, muscles, nerves and teeth.

Phthalates
Chemical compounds used as plasticisers. These compounds may cause health effects such as endocrine disruption, kidney or liver damage.

Phytochemicals (phytonutrients)
A large group of compounds produced by plants to protect them from toxins and environmental pollutants. Although not considered essential nutrients, they are believed to contain health-protecting qualities.

Picolinic acid
A metabolite from tryptophan degradation and linked to neurological inflammation.

Polychlorinated biphenyls (PCBs)
A group of biologically persistent organic compounds containing chlorine. They have a wide range of toxic effects and are linked to developmental defects, endocrine disruption, cancer.

Polyphenols
A group of chemical substances found in plants with antioxidant, anti-inflammatory properties.

Positron emission tomography (PET) scan
Produces three-dimensional, colour images of the body using radiation to provide information about the body's chemistry.

Potassium
An electrolyte and mineral that plays a major role in maintaining fluid and acid-base balance and assists in regulating neuromuscular activity.

Premenstrual syndrome (PMS)
A combination of emotional, physical, psychological and mood disturbances that occur after a woman's ovulation and typically ending with the onset of her menstrual flow.

Prostaglandins
Hormone-like substances required for a wide range of body functions, such as the contraction and relaxation of smooth muscle, the dilation and constriction of blood vessels, control of blood pressure and modulation of inflammation.

Proteins
Proteins consist of one or more chains of amino acids and are required for the structure, function and regulation of the body's cells, tissues and organs. Each protein has unique functions.

Psychosis
A mental illness seen primarily in schizophrenia and bipolar disorders. Symptoms include seeing, hearing, smelling or tasting things that are not there, paranoia and delusional thoughts.

Pyridoxine
Vitamin B6.

Quinolinic acid
A breakdown product from tryptophan degradation, which also suggests a vitamin B6 deficiency. Quniolinic acid in high levels is a neurotoxin and is linked with neurological inflammation.

Regulatory T cell
Specialised white blood cell that regulates the activity of another T cell. This process can be beneficial or harmful. There are several different types of regulatory T cells.

Saccharomyces boulardii

A tropical strain of yeast first isolated from lychee and mangosteen fruit. Classified as a probiotic, it is used to maintain and restore the natural gut flora in the treatment and prevention of gastrointestinal disorders.

Saturated fat

Type of food fat that is solid at room temperature. Most saturated fats come from animal food products, but some plant oils, such as palm and coconut oil, also contain high levels.

Schizophrenia

A complex mental health disorder characterised by hallucinations and/or delusions, personality changes, withdrawal and serious thought and speech disturbances.

Scurvy

Deficiency of ascorbic acid (vitamin C) characterised by spongy and bleeding gums, bleeding under the skin and extreme weakness.

Seasonal affective disorder (SAD)

A type of depression that tends to occur in the autumn and winter.

Secretory IgA (sIgA)

An important immunoglobulin found in the gastrointestinal tract and mucus secretions throughout the body. SIgA is our first line of defence against bacteria, food residues, fungi, parasites and viruses. Low levels are believed to be associated with allergy, autoimmune and GI diseases.

Selenium

An essential trace mineral that activates glutathione peroxidase, an antioxidant enzyme involved in the neutralisation of free radicals.

Single-photon emission computerised tomography (SPECT) scan

A type of nuclear imaging test that shows how blood flows to tissues and organs.

Spelt

An ancient grain that preceded wheat and has a higher nutritional value and mineral content.

Spirulina

A type of blue-green algae used as a dietary supplement and whole food.

Taurine

A non-essential amino acid, although it may be essential for individuals with certain diseases or nutritional concerns.

Thiamine
Vitamin B1.

Thromboxane
Member of the family of lipids known as eicosanoids. Causes blood clotting and constriction of blood vessels.

Thymus
An organ that is part of the lymphatic system, in which T lymphocytes grow and multiply. The thymus is in the chest behind the breastbone.

Trace elements
Nutrients required by plants, animals or humans in minute amounts.

Trans fats
A type of fat, formed from hydrogenation, that changes a liquid oil into a solid fat. Trans fats are found in processed foods and are now considered to be harmful to health.

Triglycerides
The chemical form in which most fat exists in food as well as in the body. Triglycerides in plasma are derived from fats eaten in foods or made in the body from other energy sources like carbohydrates. Excess levels contribute to a person's risk of heart disease.

Tryptophan
An amino acid that occurs in proteins, is essential for growth and normal metabolism and a precursor of niacin and serotonin.

Unsaturated fat
A fat that is liquid at room temperature and comes from plant foods. Can be monounsaturated or polyunsaturated.

Vanadium
A trace element important for normal cell function and development. It is thought to help maintain stable blood sugar levels.

Xenobiotic
A chemical found in an organism that is not normally produced or expected to be present, such as drugs or pollutants.

Xenohormesis
The hypothesis of how signalling molecules produced by one species (xeno), once consumed, can induce a protective response in another species during times of severe environmental stress (hormesis). It may explain how certain plant polyphenols, which indicate stress in plants, can have a beneficial effect in humans.